EFFORTLESS Back Pain Solutions

RAMIN WARAGHAI
Foreword by Dr. John Demartini

EFFORTLESS Back Pain Solutions

YOUR WAY TO A STRONG AND HEALTHY BACK

MEYER & MEYER SPORT

British Library of Cataloguing in Publication Data
A catalogue record for this book is available from the British Library

EFFORTLESS Back Pain Solutions
Maidenhead: Meyer & Meyer Sport (UK) Ltd., 2021
ISBN: 978-1-78255-207-9

Aachen, Auckland, Beirut, Cairo, Cape Town, Dubai, Hägendorf, Hong Kong, Indianapolis, Manila, Maidenhead, New Delhi, Singapore, Sydney, Tehran, Vienna

Member of the World Sport Publishers' Association (WSPA), www.w-s-p-a.org
Printed by Print Consult GmbH, Munich, Germany
Printed in Slovakia

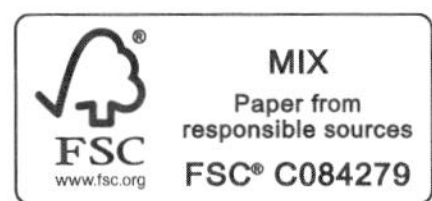

ISBN: 978-1-78255-207-9
Email: info@m-m-sports.com
www.thesportspublisher.com

CONTENTS

FOREWORD

Back pain in our western culture has traditionally been explained from a biomedical and physiological perspective. We have looked at the damage of the structures in our patients' bodies and have drawn conclusions about their pain's origin accordingly. When we realized that this approach could not always provide adequate solutions to many of our patients' painful back conditions, some of us realized that their back pain was a highly individual and sometimes internal experience. Even trying to locate an area in the brain that clearly represented the pain experience of the individual patient became, at times, a near hopeless endeavor. Today, it is more widely accepted that back pain, especially if it's chronic or recurring, has multifactorial causes, including physiological, psychological, and social causes.

In the time that I practiced as a full-time chiropractor, I was able to recognize many psychological or perceptual patterns in my patients that correlated with their specific back symptoms. Their back pain certainly was one of the more common symptoms presented, and I recognized that in many of my patients, it was accompanied by acute psychological challenges or perceived threats to what was most important to them in their lives. The body, or physiological soma, was being impacted or affected by the psyche, and the emerging back symptoms often represented feedback mechanisms to try to get the patient to return to a more balanced, prioritized, meaningful, congruent, and authentic life.

Since the body and psyche influence each other, we can impact or change ourselves physically or psychologically in order to transform our perceived levels of pain and maximize our potential. In this book, Ramin doesn't only present numerous physical exercises to reestablish muscular balance of the body, but he also gives you great psychological tips and behavioral strategies in other areas of life, which will help you to implement wiser behavior for achieving sustained back health.

In the many human behavior seminars I present around the world, I frequently experience firsthand how some individuals claim to be to struggling in their attempt to remain focused and disciplined in the daily actions required to achieve what they assume are their most important goals. The number one reason for this struggle is that they often are setting goals that are not truly important to them, and that they are injecting the views, expectations, and values of other individuals they often admire and compare themselves to, thereby setting goals that aren't truly theirs.

With the *EFFORTLESS Method*, Ramin created an approach that can help you to reclaim your inner healing power by implementing inspiring behaviors into your life which are aligned with your own highest values and beliefs. This will ultimately increase the probability of your persevering with the activities in a congruent manner that impacts inflammation and pain thresholds.

The integration of ancient wisdom and new scientific findings in different areas of life, complemented by Ramin's original ideas, makes this book a highly valuable gem. It will inspire you to find your own path to sustained back health.

–Dr. John Demartini
International bestselling author of The Values Factor

ACKNOWLEDGMENTS

The idea of writing a book about back pain had been buzzing around in my head for several years. It wasn't until my good friend and colleague, Tino Gaeding, met the sales manager at Meyer & Meyer Sport, Martina Flessenkemper, at a conference and told her about me and my project that the book idea actually took solid form. Tino, I am incredibly grateful to you for taking the initiative on my behalf that day.

But, of course, I am just as grateful to you, Mrs. Flessenkemper, for reaching out to me and giving me the opportunity to publish my ideas in this book.

Thank you to the rest of the Meyer & Meyer team who also made a decisive contribution to the completion of this book, supporting my ideas and views and even enabling me to reach an international audience with an English version of my book.

Without the support of the family, likely no author has ever managed to finish writing a book. To Mandana, Bita, Nima, Claudia, Ali: I feel deeply grateful for your great support and participation.

My friends and colleagues have also made a definitive contribution, as they have reflected on the topics and contents of the book and have supported me whenever I needed their help. Many thanks to Jonathan Sierck, Niels Kretzschmar, Emrah Coskun, Alex Woggon, Kerim Kazan, Dimitria Narcos, Andreas Skotnik, Enno Cordes, Nima Bagherzadeh, Bijan Rashidi, Juliane Mann, Gisela Krueger, Elisabeth Bilz, and Carolin Albrecht.

A special thanks goes to my mentor, Dr. John Demartini, for all his wisdom, for writing the foreword to this book, and especially for encouraging me to believe in myself.

Last but not least, I would like to thank all the great coaches and mentors from whom I was able to learn so much. They have inspired me greatly and without them and their phenomenal work this book would not have been possible.

1 INTRODUCTION TO BACK PAIN

Do you suffer from back pain, sometimes have a lumbago, or know what it's like to have constant tension in your back or neck? You're by no means alone. An estimated 80% of people in the western world experience back pain at least once in their life. Therefore, back pain is considered one of the most common widespread ailments of our time.

There is no doubt that this is justified if one considers that it is the second most common reason why people in the western world consult a doctor after the flu. Despite our constant medical progress, we cannot get the problem under control.

The main cause of back pain is our everyday life—lots of negative stress and too little movement. Evolution has not kept pace with the rapid development of the industrial age, so the human body has not yet adapted to the high amount of sitting time and the relatively little movement as well as the hectic lifestyle.

In addition, technology, such as computers, tablets, smartphones, and televisions, further facilitate our lack of movement. And the whole thing begins as a kid, when the child spends hours sitting in school, then sits in front of the TV to play computer games, and in between "hangs out" with the smartphone, while not having enough balancing movement anymore. It is not surprising that about 40% of all 14-year-olds have already experienced some type of back pain.

The need to take countermeasures against this development is probably greater than ever before. But out of all the things we're getting bombarded with nowadays, what is the right approach to take? And why should you care about your back, if you don't have any (bigger) problems yet?

Although all human beings must deal with the same laws of gravity, each one has their own individual areas of overload, which are based on the respective habits of posture and movement, injury histories, and body proportions. These may not be noticeable at first, but with time—often only after many years and in combination with other causes (will be explained in more detail in this book)—tension or even pain can develop. It makes sense to take preventive measures against these developments.

Moreover, a more balanced posture leads to more balanced breathing which leads to more balanced mental attitude. Since all systems work best when in balance, this will enable you to live your most energetic life and release your full potential. Taking specific action to bring more balance into your body will therefore help you to empower all areas of your life.

Nevertheless, if we don't take action and symptoms occur, we usually like to get rid of them as fast as possible and prefer a "quick fix," like pills or injections. However, these usually only suppress the symptoms and do not treat their real causes.

Years of unhealthy behavior and a lack of exercise should be compensated for in a few minutes (e.g., by getting a massage or adjusting the spine), and the effects should also be retained permanently without having to change any behaviors. But that's usually not the case. They may help in the short term, but after a few days, the pain returns or even worsens. You will probably not experience any sustained relief from back pain unless those methods are accompanied by increased physical activity or other long-term habit changes.

But what are those long-term habit changes, and which ones fit you best?

1.1 MY WAY TO SUSTAINED BACK HEALTH

I have suffered from recurring back pain since I was 14 years old. Consequently, I started looking for answers to this question quite early, but I couldn't even determine where the problems came from, let alone how I could relieve the pain. People repeatedly told me, that I'm not supposed to be in such pain at my age. So, I started to suppress the pain and told myself, I just have to learn to live with it. However, this thinking meant I never tackled the problem, and I ended up suffering two herniated discs 10 years later.

In December 2008, while auditioning for a possible soccer scholarship in the US, I noticed during a twist that something had happened in my lower back. When I lay down briefly after training to rest for the next afternoon session, I felt the pain in my back getting worse, and when I wanted to get up, I realized I couldn't. I was only able to walk completely bent over; I had extreme pain, and, as much as I wanted to, I couldn't play any longer. Since the coaches were only there to watch us for that day, my dream of the scholarship was over.

In addition, I had financed my studies from playing soccer and still had to pass the last practical exams of my sports studies. The timing couldn't have been more unfortunate. Even though I was still having difficulty standing up and still experiencing pain, only two weeks later, I managed to get onto the soccer field again. In competitive sports, there's always a constant battle for the spots in the team, and health is often put aside as a consequence.

About a month later, I became aware of the effects an unhealthy back can have on the rest of the body if you continue to push through the pain. I suffered severe cartilage and meniscus damage in my left knee as a result of the constant, high stresses of daily soccer practice and the many physical classes in sports studies. Today I understand that the back is connected to the rest of the body, and that an unhealthy back can also have an effect on other parts of the body, especially the knees. Similar to back pain, knee pain often results from stiff hips, and as soon as the system experiences pain, movement patterns are altered, leading to the overstraining of certain joints.

After one and a half years of rehabilitation training and two surgeries, my doctor suggested that I quit my soccer career because he was afraid the problems would get worse. He also suggested that I not become a fitness trainer, but rather should look for a more sedentary profession. He explained to me that an almost completely removed outer meniscus and such a large piece of cartilage missing in the main load zone of my knee meant that now there is bone on bone, and it would only be a matter of time before I needed an artificial knee joint.

This doctor's perspective could actually have been very counterproductive, and, if I had followed it, could have had hindering effects on my recovery and pain relief, as I will explain later.

Fortunately, it was not an option for me to surrender to this fate, so I refused to accept the diagnosis and was determined to continue living an active lifestyle. I decided not to follow the doctor's advice and instead continued training in this area outside of my sports studies.

Another big dream of mine, besides a career as a professional soccer player, was to travel the world. Due to my studies and competitive sports, however, this had never been possible for me before. In retrospect, I realized that when one door closes, another one opens. I was given the opportunity to spend a semester abroad in Santa Barbara, California, before traveling around the world for another six months.

For my master's thesis about the soccer in the US and all the further training I had to complete, I had reasons to travel again and again. These opportunities were made possible by my injuries, and I was even able to learn from and interview some of the greatest back experts in the world. These included back expert Prof. Dr. Stuart McGill, chiropractor Dr. Eric Goodman, fascia researcher Robert Schleip, and posture expert Esther Gokhale.

I really wanted to discover the true causes of back problems and what new—including traditional—training and therapy approaches there had been so far. I also dealt with topics such as nutrition, pain research, and psychosomatics. The human behavior expert Dr. John Demartini, in particular, was able to provide me with valuable knowledge about the latter.

I've also studied and tested all known therapy and training approaches such as yoga, Pilates, physiotherapy, back pain classes, and chiropractic, but I've discovered that each person has their own individual problems and deficits, so that one particular approach cannot help everyone.

Integrating various approaches and practicing a training program tailored to my functional movement deficits helped me to finally get rid of my own back problems completely.

Science is now in agreement that the real causes of back pain, especially if chronic or recurring, go far beyond our biological understanding (causes are genetics, biomechanics, age, etc.), namely that psychological (e.g., stress, fear, mood) and social factors (e.g., cultural, socioeconomical, environmental) also increase the risk for chronic back problems. From a purely biological understanding, we can't answer the question why someone has more pain on some days and less pain on others, although the physical strain substantially stays the same.

I came to the answer using the biopsychosocial model of pain used by leading experts worldwide to explain the causes of back pain, and this model will be the basis for this book. In addition to the biological aspect (e.g., damage to the spine), this model also takes into account psychological and social aspects, which can all play a role in explaining the origin of pain.

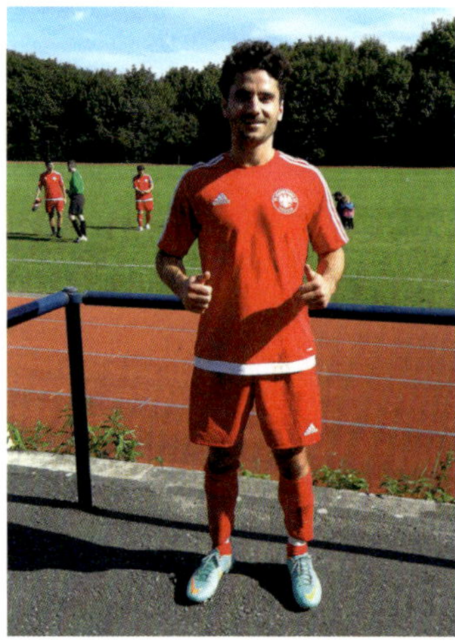

Fig. 1.1: Me after my first official soccer game in nine years

After I was able to relieve my own back problems permanently with training tailored to my functional movement deficits, it was the findings and approaches of this model that also helped me to obtain freedom from knee pain. While for years even light jogging caused me major problems, today I can play soccer without any issues, despite my missing cartilage and outer meniscus.

DISCLAIMER:

This book is not for you, if you:

- prefer to give up responsibility and blame others for your pain
- aren't open to having your beliefs about back pain challenged
- are just looking for a general exercise plan
- aren't ready to learn about your body and life
- want to stick with your belief that one must always suffer in order to achieve something
- aren't interested in learning how you could get there effortlessly

1.2 YOUR WAY TO SUSTAINED BACK HEALTH

In my 10 years as a personal trainer, training therapist, and back pain specialist helping thousands of clients suffering from back pain, it was particularly noticeable that most of them found it difficult to carry out exercises that they were supposed to do beyond our training sessions on a regular basis.

I could fully empathize with this because every time I learned something new, I tried it out, but in most cases I didn't keep it up. Hectic everyday life and all the other important things we're doing can make it difficult to change our habits. So, I asked myself: How can I convince my clients to become active beyond our training sessions and bring about changes in their everyday lives?

Besides developing a video online training program so they could do the exercises at home as well, I started training to become a health coach. The coaching approach is not like that of a personal trainer who tells the client exactly what to do, but rather is about finding suitable solutions for that specific person and their unique experiences, while considering what changes are realistic to implement in their everyday lives.

Apart from giving you effective, individualized exercises, this book also integrates the coaching approach and will make you actively participate by thinking about your life, your beliefs, and your priorities. By doing that, you won't just blindly follow what others tell you to do until giving up a few weeks later, feeling bad about yourself, and hearing yourself say over and over: "I know, I have to do some exercises, but....", or "I should start training again, but...." So, you will be required to take responsibility and create your own strategies in order to considerably increase your chances of getting sustained back health.

Since I became aware that especially prolonged or recurring back problems are always caused by many factors, I also realized that many different approaches can help. There are many different causes, so there are also many different areas in which problems can be tackled. But what is the right way for each person? And how should a plan that is individual and sustainable be designed?

I believe it should be designed in such a way that it can be implemented effortlessly, so it should be an *EFFORTLESS* plan.

Because whenever we have to spend too much effort on something, it costs us additional energy that most people just aren't willing to expend.

Therefore, the back-health plan in this book isn't about doing some exercises for a few days and then, when the initial motivation has disappeared, blaming yourself for becoming lazy and not doing the training anymore. Instead, this book is about long-term empowerment. That is why I will provide you with lots of ideas and exercises to empower you with that knowledge, but I won't tell you exactly what you have to do. Rather, I will ask you specific questions that enable you to create a realistic and individualized plan yourself, so you can find *your way* to sustained back health.

This will increase the chances of you gradually integrating the activities that suit you best into your everyday life so that you can change your habits. By doing so, you will increase your quality of life step by step, and your body will become more powerful and vital.

You will learn to resist the seduction of the victim role by taking responsibility for your health and finding ways to effortlessly solve your individual problems. With the highly topical and diverse knowledge in this book, you may even be superior to other professionals. So, I hope you're open to some new insights and suggestions and ready to get challenged on a biological, psychological, and social level.

If we consciously face challenges that make us stronger and inspire us, our body no longer exposes us to challenges that can weaken and depress us because of the tension and pain they come with.

My inspiring challenge was to research and test which exercises and methods from the individual levels of the biopsychosocial model work well and can be implemented easily.

This resulted in the *EFFORTLESS method*, which includes the following 10 parts:

Exercises

Favorite activity

Fuel

Optimizing environment

Reason determination

Treatments

Load management

Ergonomics

Stress management

Social support

In chapter 3, I will present action steps on each of these 10 areas that will give you the opportunity to help yourself. Since it will be up to you to decide which action steps you want to take, you will be able to work on your sustainable back health in your own way and at your own pace. This book is all about self-determination and initiative, to be independent from what others tell us to do or not to do. So it's mandatory to get out of the victim role, which can be assumed so quickly and easily by blaming only the circumstances for one's own problems.

Even if you're not having acute back pain, my intention is to light a spark inside of you to start mastering your back health now rather than only starting when you have already reached the point of severe pain. Prevention is often the best medicine.

Throughout, I will tell you about some of my own experiences, not to present myself as a perfect example, but rather because I hope you can gain insight if you identify with the situations.

You will learn a lot about the many causes of back pain plus some great theoretical information around all the action steps of the *EFFORTLESS method*.

This information is important in order to understand the complexity of this issue and why the individual action steps of your back-health plan will be helpful. So, I advise you not to skip this theoretical part because you might even get answers to some of the questions about back pain that have been lingering in your mind for some time.

This book is suitable for you if you either want to prevent back problems, or if you have existing problems and the causes aren't determined by your physician as "red flags" (e.g., bone fractures, infections, tumors, or nerve damage), because then you have unspecific back problems, just like approximately 90% of all cases, and the tips and exercises are most definitely suitable for you.

1.3 WHY IS THE SPINE SO IMPORTANT?

When we think about important body parts to keep healthy, we think about our heart, our lungs, our kidneys, our liver, or our brain. What we rarely think about, however, is our spine—unless, of course, we already have acute complaints. That's why only very few people are willing to do preventative work specifically for a healthy spine. In addition, this training is simply not as "sexy" as training for a slimmer figure or muscular body.

But many famous people in the past have proclaimed the importance of a healthy spine for our overall health and well-being. Thousands of years ago, the Greek philosopher Socrates said: "If you would seek health look first to the spine." Joseph Pilates, the founder of Pilates, said: "You're only as young as your spine is flexible," and in Yoga philosophy, they call the spine the "tree of life" and assert that the vitality of the spine represents the vitality of the whole being.

Without a healthy, resilient spine, our body no longer seems to be this great "tool" that gives us joy of movement and stability, but rather is a burden that we somehow learn to deal with.

This incredibly sophisticated spinal column system is a huge gift, which, despite our latest technologies, probably no engineer in the world could recreate with such precision. Its 24 free vertebrae together with the 8 to 10 fused vertebrae of the pelvis form the foundation and frame of our body at the same time.

The spine ensures that we stand upright and can also move in all directions at the same time. Besides, the spine is surrounded by all our most important organs like the heart, liver, kidneys, and lungs. It's supported by our rib cage, which helps to protect the organs and to improve its stability.

All the nerve tracts of our central nervous system run through the spinal canal and supply the entire body from there. The lumbar spine forms a stable foundation and the mobility of the other spinal parts increase the more we move up toward the head (especially in their ability to rotate). We can rotate our neck much farther than our lower back.

However, the spine doesn't make up our back alone. It is constantly interacting with other systems in our body, such as the muscular system, the fascia (connective tissue) system, or the nervous system.

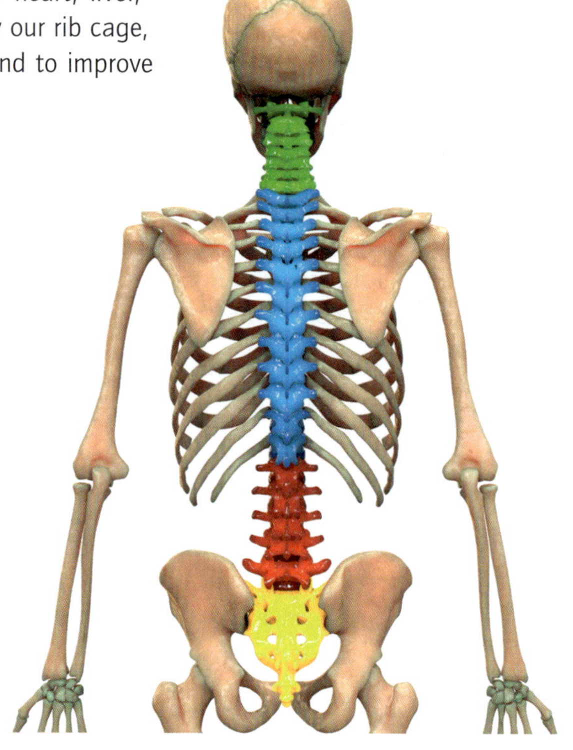

Fig. 1.2: The human spine

So, our back health not only depends on not having any spinal damage, but also on functioning in harmony with the other systems; only then can we say we have a healthy back. In many cases, even though no abnormalities are found in the spine during x-rays or MRIs, the patient still has severe pain.

All too often, the fascial system is neglected, but it has far more pain receptors than the muscular system or the spine itself. This is why more and more doctors agree that instead of an operation, in most cases, movement and exercises should first be increased to improve back health.

Even if damage is found, according to the most clinical practice guidelines, it must first be clearly ensured that there is a specific cause of the back pain before surgery is performed. Even in the case of degenerative wear and tear, the connection to the pain must first be clear before surgery so that a random diagnosis can be ruled out.

Finally, our psychological condition also plays an important role in the question of how healthy our back is. Recent studies confirm, for example, that depression is associated with back problems. Anyone who has ever had recurring back pain over a longer period of time knows all too well that in times of enormous stress, the back pain can easily flair up again.

Mental and physical condition are interrelated, so that on the other hand, something like prolonged inefficient posture can affect our breathing, which in turn affects our oxygen supply and metabolism and ultimately our mood. With chronic pain, we can quickly get into a vicious cycle, as the pain can contribute even more to a depressive mood.

In order to escape this negative spiral, it is important to understand that when we think of a healthy back, we don't only think of the spine with the individual intervertebral discs in mind, but we also consider that back health always means that the different body systems are in balance. This means that activities can help us on different levels.

In this book, our goal is to not only prevent or alleviate pain, but also to achieve a healthy back and balance in the various body systems to give more freedom of movement, vitality, and performance.

For me, freedom was and still is one of the most important things in my life. In my eyes, this also includes physical freedom, meaning the ability to move as I want, to be able to do the sport that I enjoy, and to be able to do the daily activities that are important to me.

And even if I should feel tension or pain in my back again, I would like to know exactly what I can do so that its warning signs fade.

So, if you want to live a life without restrictions and with the highest energy, freedom, and quality of life possible, it's important that you are diligent and realistic about your goals as you work through this book.

1.4 HOW EPIGENETICS GIVES BACK PERSONAL RESPONSIBILITY

When biologists announced the complete deciphering of the human genome in 2003, we were convinced that we now knew everything about how our genome builds proteins in our body. At that time, however, epigenetics (the study of changes in organisms caused by modification of gene expression rather than alteration of the genetic code itself) developed into a new field of science that would turn this theory upside down. The theory that the properties of an organism are unchangeably determined by the genetic material inherited at birth has been disproved.

In simplified terms, epigenetics was able to show that certain regions of the genome are "shut down," and that others can be transcribed more easily (into RNA for the production of proteins). Although we have certain genes in our genetic material, which genes are actually transcribed and used to produce our body's proteins ultimately depends more on us and on our living conditions than we thought.

Hence, the cells themselves regulate when and to what extent which genes are switched on or off. Why and how exactly this happens depends on our lifestyle, whether psychological traumas from childhood exist, which environmental influences we are exposed to and how we perceive them. This can epigenetically influence the development of diseases or the alteration of personality traits.

Our back health is therefore much less dependent on our genetic disposition than we previously thought. The fact that the father already had a slipped disc or chronic back problems and that it "lies in the genes" is no longer considered an excuse. It's probably not so much the bad genes, against which we can supposedly do nothing anyway, but rather behavioral patterns which we were taught or which we have copied from our parents that contribute to the transcription of genes which are either harmful or healthy for us. We should thus become aware that we, ourselves, have more responsibility for our backs than we often want to believe.

Although certain genetic predispositions, such as tissue sensitivity or bone density, determine our susceptibility to back problems, our acquired patterns of thought, behavior, and movement plus our environment and especially also our perception of it are far more important.

With the help of this book, I encourage you to consciously work on these patterns and connections and take responsibility for your health and the quality of your life back into your own hands.

By changing your environmental conditions (e.g., ergonomic workplace, health-conscious social support, stress-free environment) and your behavior (e.g., sufficient exercise, balanced mental perspectives, efficient stress management, healthy nutrition), you can have a positive influence on your genetics and not only influence your own health, but also that of your children. Even if this is not the easiest way and may entail a high level of responsibility, it's certainly all the more fulfilling and encouraging.

In this book we will work on making it as easy as possible for you.

2 THE BIOPSYCHOSOCIAL MODEL FOR BACK PAIN

2.1 THE COMPLEXITY OF BACK PROBLEMS

Before we get to the root of the true causes of back problems, we will take a moment to challenge some of the old ideas and knowledge—namely, "folk wisdom." Even new views and insights must be challenged because they don't always correspond to science, and of course individual perspective and personal experiences influence the conviction of a certain theory. I became particularly aware of this in my search for the true causes of back problems. Many experts I came across often had contrary opinions based on their own qualifications and experiences with specific client groups.

For example, some experts see constant flexion of the spine (i.e., hunchback or flat back) as the main cause of back problems in most people, whereas others see constant overstretching (i.e., hollow back or hyperlordosis) as the problem. Or one expert recommends back pain patients tighten their torsos and back muscles during movements as much as they can, and another has recognized that exactly this constant co-contraction in people with back pain is actually aggravating the problems due to the higher pressure on the intervertebral discs, and they should be taught to relax these muscles instead.

They will probably all be right in some cases, but as we will learn in this book, one method can't be used to help the total population, and only considering these physiological parameters is not sufficient to be able to explain back problems accurately. Ultimately, considering different approaches and selecting an individually suitable strategy, which make it possible to find an optimal and sustainable solution for the problems of the individual, are what count.

First, however, it should really be understood that in about 90% of cases, back pain is non-specific. This means that the pain is not attributed to any particular cause. Only about 10% have clear, immediate causes, such as damage to the nerve roots, infections, vertebral fractures, or tumors. Therefore, in the majority of cases, it is not even clear that the diagnosis made by the doctor (e.g., degenerations of the spine, disc bulges, a herniated disc, or scoliosis) corresponds clearly to the cause of the problems.

The causes of chronic or recurring back problems in particular are uncertain. A summation of studies has even shown that at least 30% of people with herniated discs don't have any back pain. In 2018, even the ***International Association for the Study of Pain*** (IASP) revised its definition of pain to: "An unpleasant sensory and emotional experience associated with, or resembling that associated with, actual or potential tissue damage."

Spinal degenerations and even a herniated disc cannot be equated with the occurrence of back pain and cannot be regarded as the sole cause of the pain. Since studies also show that they often even "spontaneously" regress after conservative treatment, rash decisions to have surgery should, in many cases, be questioned.

In order to get closer to the true causes of back problems, a holistic view is required.

2.2.1 THE BIOPSYCHOSOCIAL MODEL

One such holistic explanatory approach that has become increasingly popular in science in recent years is the **biopsychosocial model** developed by the American psychiatrist

George L. Engel (Egger, 2015). It expands our previous bio-medical understanding of the "human being as a complex machine" to a "human being as a physical-psychological being in his socio-ecological system."

So to assess the causes of a disease, it's necessary to take into account aspects at three different levels: biological, psychological, and social. All factors of each level always interact with the factors of the other two levels.

This model is based on the theory (simplified here) that health isn't the absence of disease or disorder, but a dynamic process in which the body tries every second to cope with disruptions that occur in order to ensure its proper functioning. If it's overloaded due to a lack of resources or coping skills, a "pathological" condition develops. It replaces psychosomatics to the extent that there are no longer either psychosomatic or non-psychosomatic illnesses, but each of the three levels must be considered for each illness process.

This model is now recognized by physiotherapists, medical associations, and leading back experts worldwide, especially for the causes of non-specific back problems. Universities also teach according to this model, and prospective physiotherapists nowadays always get an understanding of psychosocial causes as well.

Also the IASP stated in the enclosed notes to their new definition of pain that "pain is always a personal experience that is influenced to varying degrees by biological, psychological, and social factors."

This biopsychosocial model is also the foundation of this book, and I will present you all the different factors of those three areas to give you a holistic overview of the causes of back pain and to prove their interconnectedness.

A biological factor, be it a degeneration of the intervertebral discs, a disc bulge, or a scoliosis, can only be seen as "match," which, under unfavorable conditions (accumulated biopsychosocial factors), can ignite a fire (i.e., pain). Such biological factors are present in most of the population and are regarded as something "normal." Without the other unfavorable conditions, it can be that, as with 30% of people with herniated discs but without symptoms, fire doesn't occur. If it does, it can often be quickly extinguished by improving these unfavorable conditions alone without having to remove the match.

These unfavorable biopsychosocial factors can be psychological stress, social overload, or physical overuse. Since so many factors can play a role, it's often observed that, depending on who's looking at the problem, various causes are named. If, for example, a chiropractor looks at someone's back, he will notice the misalignment of the vertebrae and want to adjust it; a physiotherapist will instead look at the tense tissue and try to loosen it; an orthodontist will recognize that the malposition of the dentition is the cause of the problems; and a psychologist will see the initial problem in permanent stress and certain anxieties.

The human body consists of various systems, each with several specific functions that interact with each other. Some of these systems are:

- the nervous system
- the cardiovascular system
- the hormonal system
- the gastrointestinal system
- the immune system
- the muscular system
- the skeletal system
- the fascial system

Since all these systems strive for homeostasis (balance) and affect each other, disturbances in one system may cause disturbances in another. Hence, it's important to understand that a single system cannot be held solely responsible for symptoms of back pain.

The body always tries to get itself back into homeostasis, and this mechanism is called allostasis. Our body is always on our side. It's just that when the demands on it become too much due to an unhealthy lifestyle and a lot of negative stress, many systems are constantly getting out of balance, which overwhelms the body. As a result, its ways to deal with those changes become less efficient. It then needs our conscious support to change the demand that's put on it, or otherwise the allostatic load (i.e., the costs of adaptation) becomes too big (allostatic overload), creating tension or pain that alerts us to those imbalances.

The good news is that by doing things that support the body in one system can also lead to improvements in another system. So, for example, working on the elasticity of the fascial network can have a positive effect on the bones of the spinal column.

Such interactions also exist within the three levels of the biopsychosocial model. Here, psychosocial stress in particular can have negative effects on all the physical-biological systems mentioned. Often it is the combination of factors on different levels that can lead to pain. In the case of a supposedly incorrect movement, a lumbago often occurs only when we are in a very stressed state of mind at the same time. The following barrel model presented in fig. 2.1 shows how back problems are subject to an interaction of various, unfavorable causes.

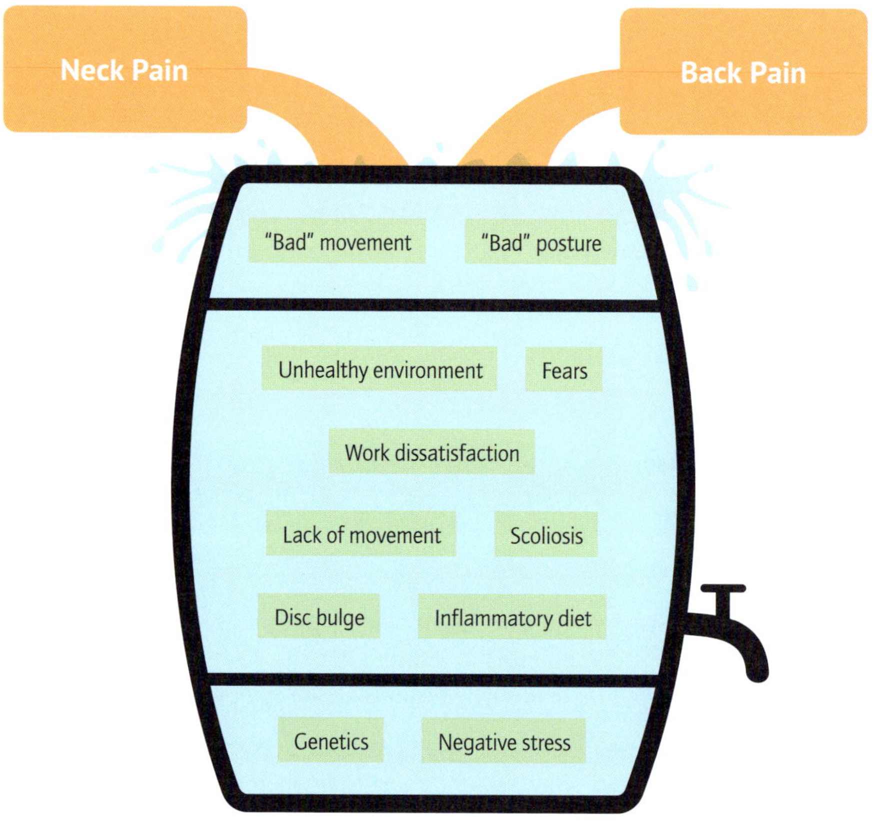

Fig. 2.1: The barrel model illustrating the causes of back pain

Imagine a barrel that is constantly filled by each of the factors of all three levels until it overflows. The overflow is equated with the triggering of a pain. Each factor increases the likelihood of developing back problems. It's unclear (and individually different) how much influence each factor has on filling the barrel, this also depends on the intensity and extent of the factor.

This model, however, makes it clear that the apparent causes of the pain, such as supposedly "incorrect" movement, are only the tip of the iceberg and by no means the only causes.

THREE LEVELS OF FACTORS FILLING THE BARREL

1. Physical-biological factors: lack of exercise, unfavorable static posture, one-sided movements, pelvic tilt, scoliosis, structural damage, inflammatory diet, dental and jaw problems, vision deficits, previous injuries, muscular imbalances, hormonal imbalances, organ dysfunctions, genetic dispositions, muscle weakness, overweight, smoking, lack of sleep, poor vital parameters, other diseases
2. Psycho-emotional factors: stress, anxiety, depression, inner conflict, dissatisfaction with work, childhood trauma
3. Social-environmental factors: difficult social relationships, workplaces not meeting ergonomic standards, unsuitable training instructions, lack of social support, unfavorable sleeping conditions, workplace-related risk factors (e.g., whole-body vibration, lifting, carrying, pulling, etc.)

As the barrel is constantly filled by the different factors, the symptoms become increasingly stronger. It may begin with slight tension, a tingling sensation, or extremities rapidly falling asleep. Then there are increased feelings of tiredness and listlessness; finally, the back hurts, acutely (e.g., after a lumbago), recurrently, or even permanently.

In the case of back problems, our body's warning signals are still pretty quiet at the beginning. But if we don't change anything to prevent the accumulation of factors, those signals become louder and louder, and the biological factors (or the "match") get closer and closer to the edge.

If you then get a lumbago, as in the previous example, it was not only the one unfavorable movement that led to the pain, but the combination of factors such as stress, an unhealthy diet, and lack of exercise, which had already filled the barrel before. The fuller it is, the more susceptible we are to all pain. The "match" then only determines exactly where the pain occurs.

If there is a lot of "match" and our barrel gets full to the point of overflowing, we quickly feel it in the neck, then in the lower back, and then there are also shoulder and knee problems. It may seem to us in this case that we are "broken" everywhere, but in reality, our barrel is too full, meaning we have let those factors accumulate to the point of acute pain.

When you look at the different layers of the barrel what do you think are the proportions of the different factors in your case? Is the most influential area the physical-biological because you know your body has been under strain and has accumulated a lot of "lit matches"? The psycho-emotional because you are currently highly stressed and are worried because of your symptoms? Or do you feel socially isolated or believe that your environment doesn't really facilitate a healthy lifestyle?

It's unique to every person, and there is no right or wrong. Be aware of which parts have the greatest impact on your health and bear that in mind as later on you will want to select the right action steps that will help you empty your barrel.

Fortunately, the barrel also has a drain (see fig. 2.2) through which it can be emptied. So the accumulated factors can be counteracted by, for example, moving more, individualizing back training and fascia training, improving posture and movement habits, managing stress, getting treatments, following anti-inflammatory nutrition, and using relaxation techniques and psychotherapy.

The emptier the barrel, the less likely we are to suffer pain and the greater our vitality, quality of life, and performance.

So, it makes sense to not only empty the barrel as much as possible in order to avoid pain, but also to make better use of our potential and live the way we would wish to. Emptying the barrel is also important, because only avoiding pain often doesn't motivate us enough to work on our health permanently.

Health is a process in which we want to keep our barrels as empty as possible and strengthen our health resources by constantly creating balance in the various body systems. This model may sound pretty complex, but it's an explanation for the questions that back pain sufferers keep asking themselves, such as: "Why are there days when I notice the pain less and then again days when the pain is unbearable, although I didn't move any differently than usual?" The answer is simple: Because the barrel was fuller.

So not only one physical-biological factor alone can be responsible, because then there wouldn't be these daily fluctuations of pain intensity. It's all biopsychosocial factors that fill the barrel more on one day and less on another. Although with this model we might think that getting a lasting healthy back would be very complicated and exhausting, you will see in chapter 3 how to do this effortlessly by learning to empty your barrel with individualized strategies.

When need to change our perspective from thinking that there is nothing we can do because we have so many pains, aches, and imbalances to seeing it as potential for us to empty the bucket and live a more energetic and fulfilling life; changing this perspective is key in this approach. So I hope you won't get too overwhelmed by all the various factors, because you will learn great methods that will help you to deal with all of them.

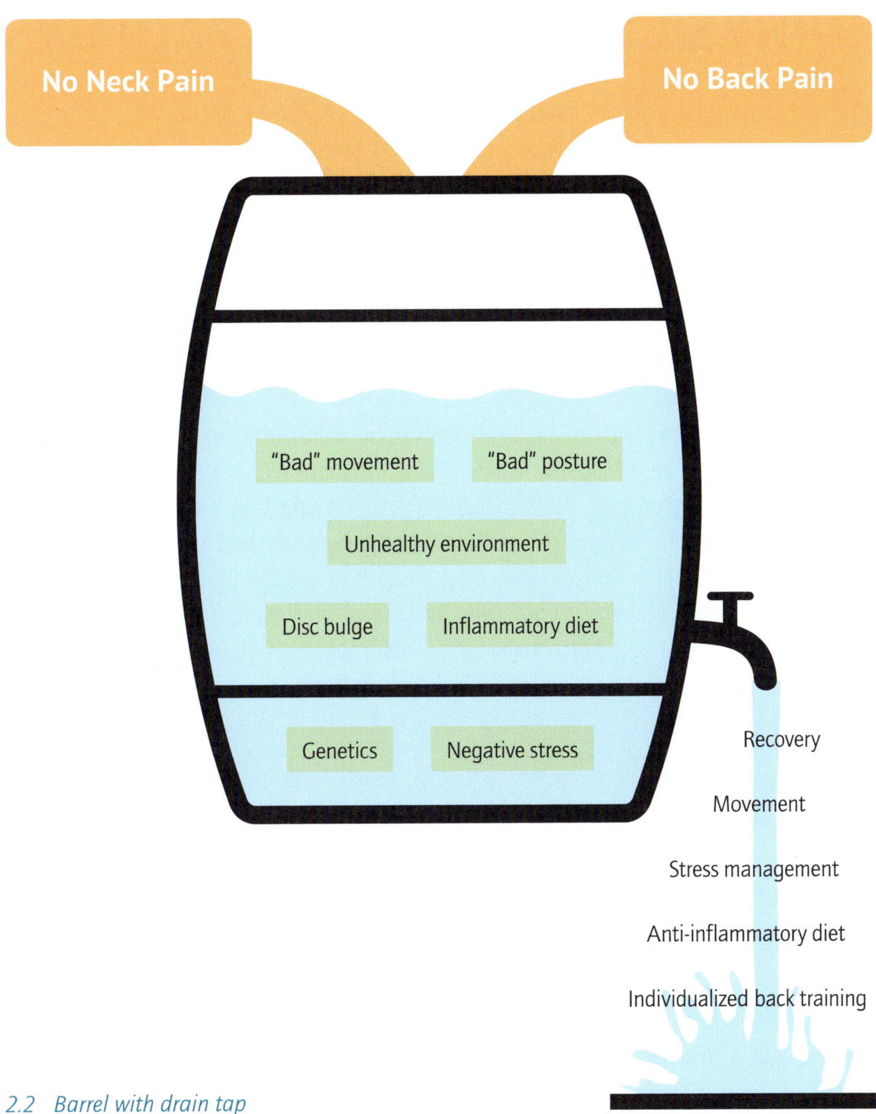

Fig. 2.2 Barrel with drain tap

2.2 PHYSICAL-BIOLOGICAL FACTORS

The physical-biological factors seem to be what fill our barrel fastest as all disorders of the structures and systems of our body can lead to them. They are crucial in determining the location of pain or tension, but, as mentioned, they cannot be identified as a clear cause in about 90% of back pain.

Nevertheless, many doctors, physiotherapists, and trainers are still convinced that pain can only be explained in a biomedical way, and they reject the important influence of psychosocial factors. Even the latest scientific findings on the biology of the body increasingly point toward interaction with psychosocial factors.

This is confirmed by the fields of fascia research, pain therapy, and respiratory sciences, which we will examine more closely in the following sections. In all these areas, it's clear that the causes and effects of the individual factors cannot be clearly determined, but rather there's a constant interaction between the biological and the psychosocial area. Whether the psychosocial factors arise first and then create biological factors or vice versa is basically the "chicken or egg" question. You can't really say for certain because they're both developing simultaneously. So in this book, we will just look at their mutual influences and leave it to you to decide which ones you wish to address.

2.2.1 DIAGNOSES

We're all about getting diagnoses these days. Until we know exactly what we have, we can't sleep peacefully. We even often try to self-diagnose. We google our symptoms and find the most horrible pictures and reports and then are convinced that is probably what we have. But are diagnoses important for our recovery after all?

Regarding back problems, they are important in only a few cases (the 10% mentioned previously). In the other 90% of cases, where there are no suspicious red flags, and the causes are non-specific, the diagnosis is rather secondary. More important in these cases is the question: How full is our barrel?

The diagnosis could be interesting for a physiotherapist, osteopath, or training therapist, so that he or she can arrange treatment or training suggestions accordingly. For us and our recovery, however, it doesn't play a prominent role if red flags can be excluded.

A diagnosis that wear and tear of the spine, a herniated disc, or something similar is present can certainly make us worry. After all, who wants to hear that their spine has aged or is damaged? That's why Lorimer Moseley and David Butler, two of Australia's best-known pain specialists, warn against giving too much importance to diagnoses (Butler, 2016). The majority of the "matches" found represents things that are completely normal for most people anyway. They can contribute to filling the barrel, but they don't mean that we ever have to have pain at all.

Since in about 90% of all acute back problems, the pain disappears by itself within the first four to six weeks, imaging techniques should only be used if pain persists beyond this time period (or when red flags are suspected), according to most clinical practice guidelines. In reality, though, they are often used much earlier to come up with an acceptable explanation for the pain. Part of why that is happening is because we insist on getting a precise diagnosis which in 90% of the cases just isn't possible and wouldn't even tell us the whole story anyway.

In addition, a diagnosis is not always accurate. Frequently one doctor makes a diagnosis that another doctor wouldn't. Upon receiving a diagnosis, we then think we know what's wrong and are reassured—or if our worst fear has really come true, we worry even more—but, on the one hand, the diagnosis is not even 100% certain, and, on the other hand, knowing it is often irrelevant for our recovery anyway. In fact, the diagnosis encourages our urge to take on the comfortable victim role because then we can blame our unfortunate physical circumstances for our pain rather than tackling the issues that led to this pain (our filled barrel). But if we accept this victim role, the probability that our back problems will become chronic is at its highest.

So however strong and real our pain may feel, it can often be beneficial (if "red flags" have been excluded) for us to concentrate more on emptying the barrel instead of trying to get a diagnosis at all costs.

I was in the comfortable position of the victim role for years. I was able to tell everyone how bad it was for me to have two herniated discs at the age of 23. Again and again, I heard responses like: "At your age? That's really bad!" or "A herniated disc? Soccer really destroyed your body."

While at the beginning I lapped up the sympathy, after I learned about the true causes of back problems, I started to say, "Well, many people have herniated discs! It's nothing out of the ordinary, and it doesn't cause me any problems."

The (hard) truth is, in almost every adult in our western world, signs of wear and tear can be found in various joints of the body if they're examined in detail. If you now have pain and go to the doctor with it, the probability is high that the doctor will find something, allocate it to the existing pain, and consequently treat it or operate on it. In many cases, however, the pain would probably have gone away without treatment if the barrel had been emptied.

However, this doesn't mean that the "match" should never be blown out if there is a possibility and if it's considered acutely necessary. The question is, what are the consequences? And can the condition also be improved to the same extent or even more promisingly by emptying the barrel through accurate training, chiropractic adjustment, or by eliminating any of the other contributing factors?

In many cases, the more reasonable approach would be to trust in the strength of the body, to deal with the alleged damages, and to support the body as much as possible by emptying the barrel.

In an ideal world, of course, we wouldn't want all of the wear and tear to be created in the first place, but unless we consciously start working on balancing our body at a young age, it's quite unrealistic to assume we wouldn't have any. Still, I highly recommend adopting a perspective that considers long-term physiological changes instead of short-term pain fixes, whether you're already in pain or you want to prevent yourself from ever being in pain.

2.2.2 COMPENSATORY PATTERNS

There are also numerous cases in which a back-pain sufferer wants to be diagnosed, but the doctor wasn't able to find anything in the imaging procedures. The patient is often sent home afterwards and is told that the pain is only psychological, meaning it only exists in the head. In (almost) all cases, psychological causes are accompanied by biological causes as well.

With the help of a detailed analysis and the right tests, compensatory patterns (less efficient patterns the body uses to perform motions when mobility or stability are not sufficient) can be found in these cases, which are associated with mobility deficits, muscle weaknesses, and muscle imbalances, which could've caused overloading of the respective structures. They may not be diagnosable with imaging, but they are still to be regarded as a "match."

Often, either the time isn't taken to carry out the necessary tests, or competence is lacking. Canadian back expert Dr. Stuart McGill (2015), for example, performs specific tests for up to three hours to find out what motion, posture, and load triggers the pain. According to his statements, he almost always finds a physical reason for overload in the form of compensatory patterns or pain-triggering movements. Consequently, he's a critic of purely psychological explanations of back pain.

The same holds true for the experiences we made with our online program in which we used a seven-exercise self-test prior to training in which we looked for imbalances in mobility and stability that usually lead to those compensations. From thousands of participants, almost no one was able to pass all the tests, which means that almost every participant had a "match" somewhere. But where do these compensatory movements come from anyway?

In our early developmental phases, we learned at some point to move efficiently, meaning with the lowest energy consumption and wear (unless there were developmental impairments due to traumas or genetic deformities). We had excellent mobility and moved freely, without problems.

A good example of this is how a child picks something up with optimal technique or plays with something in front of him, remaining in a deep squat position (see fig. 2.3) for an extended period without any problems, which many adults in our western societies cannot even hold for a few seconds.

Through our modern lifestyle with all its prolonged sitting, one-sided sports, as well as through old injuries, traumas, and bad role models who moved inefficiently themselves, we have acquired compensatory patterns. These compensations have a particularly important role: They primarily guarantee our survival, as they preserve our main functions, such as our senses of sight and our emotions. In order to also protect us from injuries and minimize future pain, our body does everything in its power and uses compensatory movements to avoid danger.

For decades, the many stresses and strains of everyday life were put aside without any problems, and the entire body learned in an incredible way how it can compensate even better. It's not too ambitious to say that the body's compensations are a real miracle.

However, the human body is such a finely tuned system that the muscles can perform optimally in the balance between strength and elasticity. But if a certain demand knocks this system out of balance, then there are altered loads on the joints, which the body then must compensate for in other segments. This leads to a loss of energy during movements and overloading of the overstrained muscles as well as the surrounding passive structures, such as the bones, joints, or ligaments.

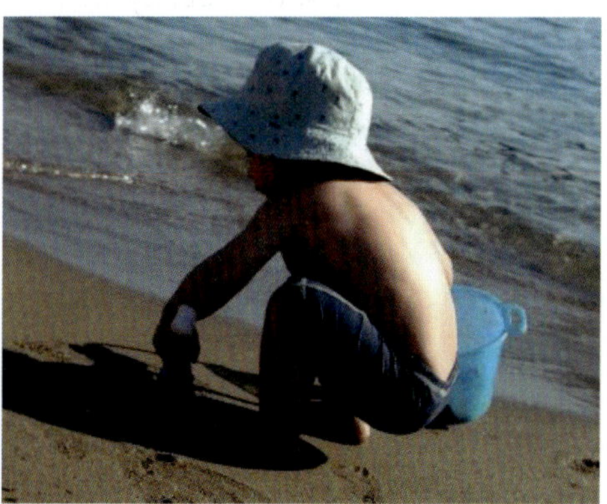

Fig. 2.3: Children easily play in deep squat positions

The body remains strong and resistant, but it does not work as efficiently as before, and with time or increased stress, the overloaded structures can become noticeable.

If breathing difficulties occur, for example, the neck muscles are used more frequently to help the diaphragm (the main breathing muscles) get air into the lungs by pulling up the shoulders. If this becomes a habit, the neck muscles become overloaded, and neck tension and other problems can develop.

With scoliosis (lateral curvature of the spine), the body must compensate in the opposite direction so that the person can continue to look straight ahead, otherwise their sense of balance would be massively disturbed. To accomplish this, the body tilts the head, for example, slightly to the opposite side, whereby one shoulder is higher, and the neck muscles of this side can become tense.

All those compensations filling the barrel often go unnoticed. If other biopsychosocial factors are added, the back will at some point begin to demand changes from us. It's still on our side; it just needs our conscious support.

The body's problem is that it has become so accustomed to these compensations that it keeps them until the trigger for them has disappeared. Often not even then, because it needs another movement pattern to guarantee the respective function. It can either use old patterns it learned in childhood or completely new ones if they're specifically trained.

Remaining in certain positions for long periods of time can also affect our posture. If, over the years, we've become accustomed to sitting bent over and only rarely adjust our posture, a kyphosis (hunchback) can develop. However, changes in our posture can also be caused by psychological moods. Factors such as stress, depression, worry, or anxiety can certainly influence our posture. For example, if you feel overwhelmed or anxious, you tend to lower your head and round your upper back. Or if you feel the need to constantly assert yourself, you might push your chest out so far that you create a reinforced arched back. On the other hand, recent studies also show that a bent posture can promote depressive states, which confirms the interaction of biological and psychosocial factors.

Back then, I would have counted myself in the hunchback category because I was a rather shy boy who, in order to hide, often lowered his head to make himself small. In addition, I had pretty immobile hips—typical for soccer players—which facilitated lots of compensations in my lower back.

One of the top physiotherapists in the world, American Shirley Sahrmann (2001), calls these compensations "movement impairments" and asserts that back problems often arise when we constantly compensate from the back (and especially from the lumbar spine), because our hips no longer participate in movements properly. This leads to hypermobility (overly mobile) of the spine, exactly in the area where we compensate the most (see fig. 2.4), causing tissue injury and degeneration. When asked "what's the most important thing you've identified in your 50 years of practicing?" Sahrmann said, "It's that the body takes the path of least resistance. It hurts where it moves, and it moves where it's the easiest to move." So, also in the spine, you'll move mostly in the area that is the most flexible.

Basically, the spine, as we all know, should be sufficiently flexible. However, the hips and shoulder girdles should always be at least as mobile, otherwise there's a high probability that we will compensate for this in other areas. Only when each segment of the spine has its optimal mobility, without one being hyper- or hypomobile due to compensation, are truly efficient movements of the spine possible. This means that the lumbar spine can, of course, be hypomobile in many cases as well, and compensations may then occur in the thoracic spine, causing problems there.

My only strategy against back pain at that time was to stretch the lumbar spine. Although this felt good, it made this hypermobile segment even more unstable in the long term, while my hips remained immobile. This circumstance probably contributed to my two herniated discs. Dr. Stuart McGill (2015) sees the "neurological phenomenon of the stretch reflex" as the reason for the temporarily pleasant feeling caused by the stretching. Although it gives you 15 to 20 minutes of analgesia, which feels good, it's often only a short-term solution that makes you think you need to do it over and over.

Though such short-term solutions can sometimes be useful in order to enable movement again, they can also have counterproductive long-term consequences, as happened in my case. Because my lumbar spine became more and more unstable, the pain kept coming back.

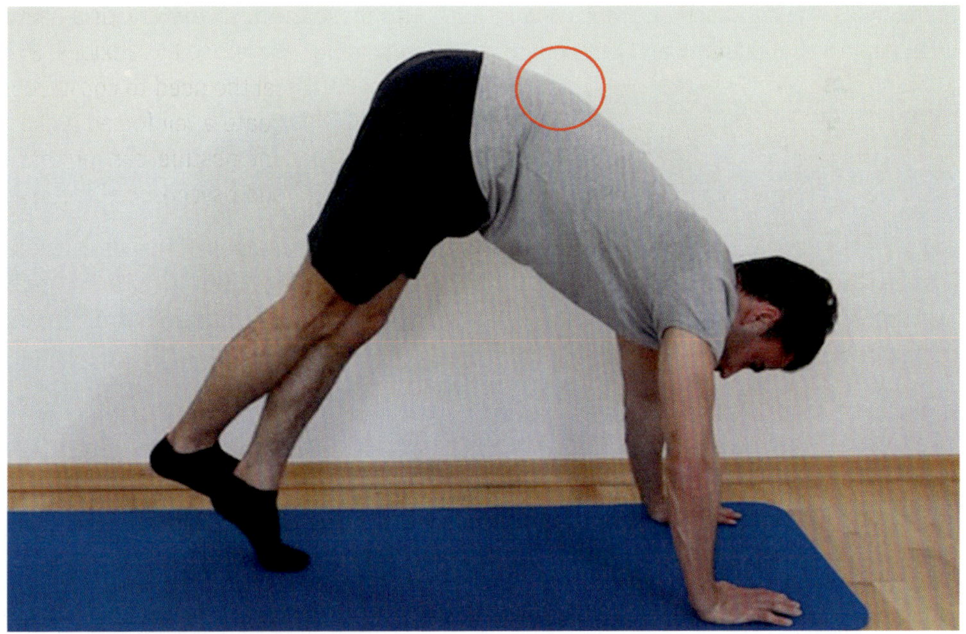

Fig. 2.4: Compensation in the lower back

As you can see in fig. 2.4, my body compensated at a certain point in the lower back due to the lack of mobility in my hamstrings, calves, and glutes.

Finding out where there are deficits in mobility and how passive structures are overloaded by possible compensatory patterns before then increasing mobility in the areas that need it and creating more efficient movement patterns that eliminate the compensatory movements is a reasonable strategy to counteract these overloads in the long term. In chapter 3 we will conduct simple self-tests to identify your most important mobility deficits, so that you can then select the exercises that minimize your individual compensations best.

2.2.3 PAIN-TRIGGERING FASCIAL NETWORK

"Fascia" has been on everyone's lips for several years now, especially in the fitness sector, and in rehabilitation it's become increasingly important. And rightly so, since science is gaining more and more insight into these fascinating connective tissue structures, and the resulting methods for (self-) treatment are helping numerous people.

The way we treat fascia with foam rollers, tennis balls, and so on may be a temporary trend, but knowledge about fascia will continue to be important for our understanding of the body. This is because discoveries and insights into the many functions of fascia allow us to explain the anatomy and physiology of our body in new ways.

But what exactly is fascia? Fascia are woven structures, such as ligaments, tendons, or cartilage, that form a three-dimensional network, connecting the entire body in fascia lines from the big toe to the forehead; it envelops muscles, joints, bones, and organs in several layers. Because fascia connects the entire body, researchers have now decided to call it the fascial network. This system allows the individual areas of our body to be supplied with fluid, nutrients, and oxygen. The fascial network is both flexible and tear resistant. It forms a functional network together with the muscles, transferring forces from muscle to muscle and absorbing enormous shocks. The fascial network is also often referred to as the myofascial network and its myofascial chains.

To envision of bodies' facial networks, you should visualize a mandarin that's been peeled, and the white threads pulled apart. These white threads are like having parts of the fascial system in your hand (see fig. 2.5).

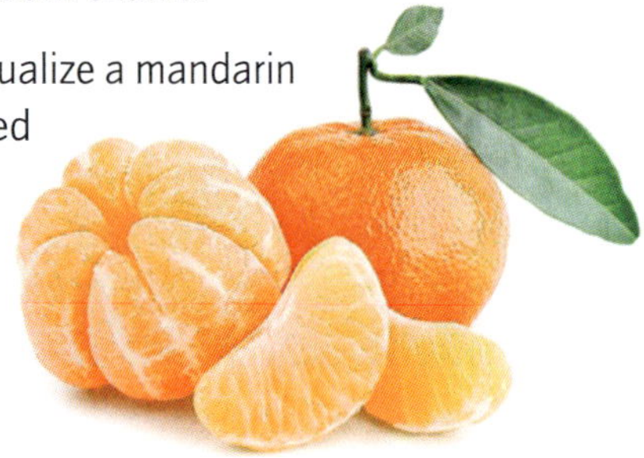

Fig. 2.5: Fascia of a mandarin.
Each flesh chamber of the mandarin, like the muscles in our body, is surrounded by fascia.

BUT WHAT DOES FASCIA HAVE TO DO WITH OUR BACK PAIN?

According to Robert Schleip (2014), a world-renown German fascia researcher, the fascial system (if the subcutaneous connective tissue, the intramuscular connective tissue, and the joint capsules are included) can be described as an independent sense organ—thus as our sixth sense—because it possesses several million nerves and is more richly innervated than the sense of sight. Our functional, inner-body perception (proprioception) is controlled via this sense organ. Thanks to it, we know, for example, whether one shoulder is higher than the other or whether we're sitting with an arched back.

Due to lack of movement in particular, permanent and one-sided postures, or numerous compensatory movements, the fascial network is no longer supplied with sufficient fluid; as a result, its structures become disorganized, matted, and the individual fascial layers stick together.

This also disturbs our proprioception. We no longer realize that we're sitting in a slouched or overarched position; our head is moving forward when staring at the computer screen for too long; or that we're lifting one arm way higher when bringing the hands above the head. But those imbalances slowly but surely lead to even greater tension. Numerous pain receptors of the fascial system send signals to our brain, which are intended to cause sensations of tension or pain in order to bring those imbalances to our attention.

The large dorsal fascia (thoracolumbar fascia) is particularly relevant for back pain sufferers, as it extends over the entire lumbar vertebra area and parts of the thoracic vertebra area, including many muscle connections and pain receptors. Studies show that in people with chronic low back pain, the fascia in that area is thicker and its structure is more disorganized.

By knowing this, it may also be possible to explain where the pain signals come from in back pain sufferers with no clear diagnosis.

The latest findings indicate that the fascial system also reacts to stress. Its condition is dependent on the biochemical environment they're in as well. Distress leads to an acid pH value, whereby the fascia contracts and hardens more quickly, triggering pain signals.

Because of these interactions with psychological factors, the physical changes in the lumbar fascia in people with back pain are not necessarily the causes of chronic back pain, but rather they can be the effects of psychological distress. Whatever the case may be, learning more about the fascial system can help us understand from where the pain signals in 90% of people with unspecific back pain originate, and focusing on treating the fascial network offers promising opportunities to alleviate the pain.

Moreover, these new findings about the fascial network prove how much biological factors interact with psychosocial factors.

2.2.4 LACK OF EXERCISE

We live in a time in which physical labor is becoming less important which means movement has decreased in a way that has not happened before. However, this not only causes several lifestyle diseases (e.g., obesity, diabetes, heart disease), but also back pain in particular. Most people, especially in the western world, don't achieve the recommended 10,000 steps a day. The world average lies at about half that. Plus, the World Health Organization (WHO) recommends adults aged 18 to 64 to do a minimum of 150 minutes of moderate aerobic exercise plus two sessions of weight training every week in order to live a healthy life. Most people don't make these numbers either.

If we compare ourselves with people from the Stone Age, we should notice that, despite the significantly higher physical strain, they experienced degenerative joint changes less frequently than we do today. One of the reasons for this is that our cartilage and our intervertebral discs need movement to be nourished, and they were moving way more than we do today.

Movement is a natural way to empty our barrel because of its vast health-promoting effects. Movement not only strengthens the muscles, bones, and joints and keeps intervertebral discs healthy, but it also promotes blood circulation, supplying our body's complete fascial system with fluid and nutrients. This helps to better inhibit inflammation, prevent pain hypersensitivity, and remove waste products. It's important to note that while even light endurance training that gets us out of breath or sports for which our heartbeat only reaches about 120-140 bpm would be enough for these positive effects, the key is that the activities must be done voluntarily.

In addition, exercise strengthens the immune system, releases endorphins that improve our mood, and increases our energy levels. Exercise can decrease heightened stress levels, lower the risk of depression and anxiety disorders, improve movement patterns and coordination, and lead to weight loss.

Movement also helps to prevent chronic complaints. So even just a few days after lumbago or a slipped disc occurs, it's very important to get moving again and carry out daily activities as much as possible.

Because of all these health-promoting effects, most experts today agree that movement and exercise—whether it's walking, jogging, swimming, or a particular sport—are key to emptying the barrel.

You don't even need to play a specific sport or have an exercise regimen. If we simply increase the amount of everyday movement, you also experience these health-promoting effects. These everyday movements are called *Non-Exercise Activity Thermogenesis, or more simply, NEAT activities*. These include all movements that aren't specifically part of a sport or exercise regimen. In chapter 3, you'll get some ideas on how you can integrate some more NEAT activities into your everyday life.

2.2.5 PROLONGED AND ONE-SIDED POSTURES IN EVERYDAY LIFE

To get a healthy back, training a few hours a week can be quite helpful. However, if in the remaining 160-plus hours our behavior involves many unfavorable habits, those positive effects can be lost again. It's become normal in our western world to sit for 7 to 10 hours a day. That's about half the time we're awake. If unfavorable behaviors are not changed here, the likelihood the barrel will fill up is very good.

The most unfavorable behavior we've adopted is sitting for several hours at a time without moving in any way. In addition, we're "pushed" into a rather slumped posture from an early age. From poor child seats, new media such as smartphones, tablet, or laptops to non-ergonomic workplaces in schools, our environment is characterized by conditions that encourage rounding the spine; we very quickly acquire our favorite compensatory slumped sitting position. Instructions such as: "Sit up straight" or "puff out your chest and pull your shoulder blades together" are not useful approaches to counteract this. They usually promote an overextended posture (arched back) and can also lead to tension and back problems if the child remains in this position for long periods of time.

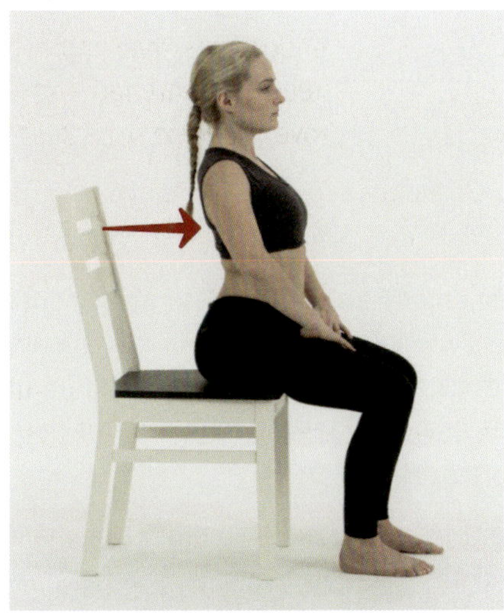

Fig. 2.6: Overextended sitting posture

Without a doubt, the topic of posture has been controversially discussed in recent years. Sitting upright has been frowned upon. Instead, only one thing is recommended here—movement.

Dynamic sitting (i.e., frequently changing the sitting position to avoid permanent tension) is currently the number one recommendation of many back experts. Not only do many people like to remain in their most comfortable sitting position, but this is often the position that triggered the back pain in the first place. Consciously integrating dynamic sitting into everyday life can provide pain relief. In that regard, there are no "right" or "wrong" sitting positions as the next sitting position is always the best.

Although the current state of research confirms this, and our body posture is generally assigned a subordinate role in explaining the causes of back pain, many traditional approaches, which, despite all trends, are still relevant, show that targeted improvement of posture and movement patterns can help people with back problems. These methods include the Alexander Technique, Gokhale Method, or Ismakogy.

According to these, we can make our postures more efficient and counteract overloads. The more balanced the posture, the less energy lost in the fight against gravity. With all its surrounding muscles and fascia, the spine is a physically sophisticated system that doesn't need much muscle tension to hold itself upright when it's in its neutral position. (Note: Every person's "neutral" is different.)

Balancing the tension of muscles and fascia on the front and back of the body provides stability without over activating one side. Therefore, in this position there's less stress or wear.

Optimally stacking various segments of the body with the spine in its neutral position can also lead to an improvement in mental conditions, less fatigue, more self-confidence (testosterone levels rise, cortisol levels fall), as well as organs and respiratory and digestive systems that function better. Since all of this can contribute to emptying the barrel, there are at least a number of secondary advantages in optimizing the posture which can be of decisive help.

When sitting with the spine in neutral position, there's an additional advantage that bridges the gap to dynamic sitting. From an upright sitting position, there is a greater chance that we move more. People whose predominant sitting position is slouched tend to change their sitting position much less often than people attempting to sitting upright, which in my view further justifies the attempt to sit in an upright position with the spine in its neutral position.

Ultimately, if we remain in any position (even the neutral one) long enough, no matter if it's sitting, standing, or lying down, our tissue will not be properly supplied with blood, which results in overloading and rising tension. Consequently, regular movement is extremely important.

But what about the posture of our everyday movements? Can we do these movements "incorrectly?" The answer is no! There are no "bad" or "wrong" movements. All movements that our body can perform are basically healthy. If we move versatilely, meaning in all directions and with the help of different techniques and joint angles, then the frowned-on forward bend with a round back, for example, is no problem at all.

On the contrary, our fascia network needs movement in all directions in order to remain healthy and robust. Often, however, we're still told that we must always bend with a straight back when picking something up from the floor, for example, as this lowers the strain on the back. While this may well be biomechanically correct, according to our current understanding of the body, it does present a problem. We don't bring this important lumbar fascia under tension enough anymore, so it becomes weaker and more vulnerable to injury and pain.

If we're so stressed that we don't pay attention to a perfect bend with a straight back (which happens more often than we think), our lumbar fascia is no longer prepared for this sudden, strong strain and becomes extremely irritated, sending out a strong pain signal (as in a lumbago).

In this case, the doctor would say, "I warned you never to round your back," and feels confirmed in his theory. The reality of our everyday life, however, is that it's often impossible to keep our backs straight at all times; we cannot be so conscious in our everyday life as to always pay attention to it. With the new knowledge about fascia, it now becomes clear that this is not even necessary, rethinking this idea would make sense.

All movement is healthy, except when there's a single, inefficient movement pattern in which we repeatedly load the same part of the spine (i.e., compensations), and we don't have a wide range of alternative movements available.

Just as habitually remaining in a slumped sitting posture can lead to overload, so, too, can constantly repeating movements with individual compensatory patterns in everyday life. And while back pain sufferers often remain in their pain-triggering sitting postures, they also move in the pain-promoting movement patterns until they feel pain.

2.2.6 COMPENSATORY BREATHING

When it comes to movement, breathing must not be forgotten either. Why? Because it's the most important of all our movements. Without it, we could not live. The first movement we make when we're born is to expand our chest so that we can inhale. If we consider that we inhale and exhale up to 22,000 times a day and that countless joints and muscles are involved, then it becomes clear why breathing is so important for the functioning of our body. Since our breathing is one of the main functions of our body, almost all other compensations can be traced back to it. It's not for nothing that so much value is placed on breathing in yoga, Qigong, or martial arts.

Our breathing primarily ensures that we can absorb sufficient oxygen and release carbon dioxide. This regulates our pH value, and the cells can use the oxygen to provide energy. Distress, injuries, illnesses, a permanently inefficient posture, or unhealthy eating habits lead to a loss of breathing efficiency because our body has to find ways to compensate.

However, those compensations often develop physiologically as well as psychosocially without us even noticing anything.

Probably the most common compensation is the tendency to hyperventilate (i.e., when we breathe very shallowly and too often). While this may be necessary, for example, in dangerous situations or during sports, when this stress breathing becomes regular, our sympathetic nervous system is permanently active, while the parasympathetic system remains deactivated. As a result, our muscles are constantly tense, we can no longer recover optimally, we sleep poorly, and we react more sensitively to stressors. Therefore, the biggest problem isn't that we're not breathing deeply enough and not getting enough oxygen, but instead we're breathing too much.

On the biomechanical level, this stress respiration means our diaphragm is no longer properly activated. The diaphragm is the main breathing musculature in our body and makes sure we can suck air into our lungs. If it doesn't work properly, other muscles must compensate for it, including movement of other joints.

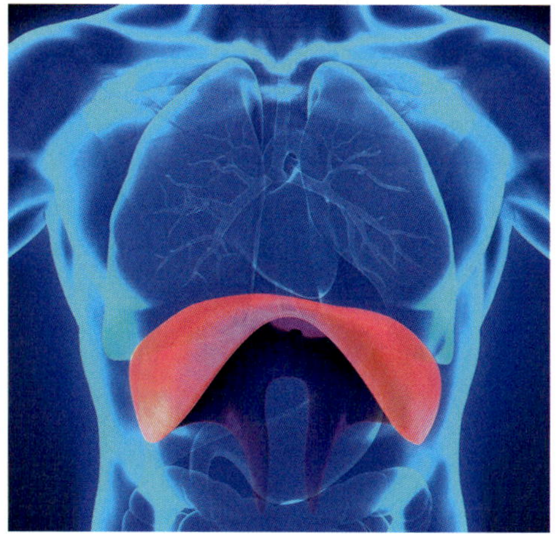

Fig. 2.7: Our most important respiratory muscle: the diaphragm

A normal inhalation pattern has three phases:

1. The pelvic floor and abdomen expand.
2. The rib cage expands.
3. Finally, the shoulders lift slightly.

One typical compensatory pattern that can be observed is breathing mainly by pulling up the shoulders, skipping the first two phases. Depending on intensity and duration, this compensation can overload the neck muscles. Not only does a tense neck result, but there are also changes in the complete stability of the spine. Due to the reduced activity of the diaphragm muscles, muscles around the thorax are shortened, and the ribs become too stiff to move, whereas they're supposed to move in almost every direction our upper body does. Sliding the chest forward and reinforcing the lordosis (arched back) is only one of the many counterproductive consequences.

Because of this negative spiral set in motion by the loss of optimal diaphragm breathing, activating diaphragm is the main goal of almost all breathing exercises. This type of breathing is oftentimes taught as "belly breathing," only breathing into the belly can also be a dysfunctional pattern since the other two phases are still neglected. If we never really expand our ribcage in our breathing patterns, it will become tense and lose its mobility, and the thoracic spine will no longer be able to extend. It might make sense to teach a shoulder-breathing person to breath into his belly and vice versa, but ultimately, we want to make sure that all three phases are used in every inhalation pattern. In addition, many people breathe mainly through the mouth, nut nose breathing has a number of advantages over mouth breathing. It filters, warms, and humidifies the air and due to the longer airways to the lungs; we tend to inhale less often during nasal breathing, which counteracts the hyperventilation compensation described previously.

Just like with the other biological factors, there's also a strong interaction with the psychosocial area in respiration. If we perceive the outside world very emotionally (e.g., with stress or fear), our breathing patterns change. We get scared and hold our breath or hyperventilate as a result. On the other hand, if we breathe inefficiently or can't breathe deeply enough because of restrictions in our body, we become more stressed and afraid, and we perceive the outside world more emotionally. Breathing exercises therefore often aim to ensure relaxation and serenity by activating the parasympathetic nervous system. Conversely, targeted hyperventilating—similar to the *Basthrika* breathing technique in Yoga—is also often used to activate the sympathetic nervous system to raise energy levels prior to an activity.

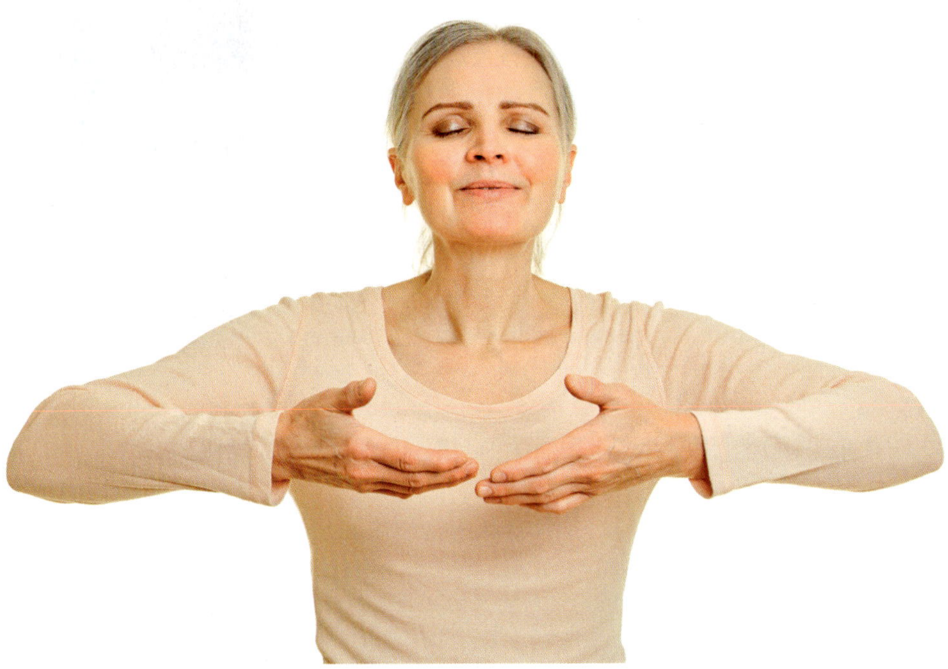

Fig. 2.8.: For efficient breathing, the diaphragm should be activated and the nose used.

2.2.7 POOR NUTRITION

Usually when we search for the causes of inflammation, we look at injuries, infections, or stress. More and more people nowadays realize that a poor diet can also cause inflammation. When we treat ourselves in the morning to a tasty croissant or muffin and a coffee, the inflammatory process already begins.

We may not necessarily feel it right after eating, but we will if we make such a breakfast a habit. Over time, if we consume more inflammatory foods and not enough anti-inflammatory foods like vegetables, fruits, or fish, the many small sources of inflammation will fill our barrels more and more.

This is because inflammatory foods, such as sugar, hardened fats, or dark meat, ensure a low (acidic) pH value in our body. Similar to stress, the acidic pH value created by inflammatory foods affects the health of our fascia. In an acidic environment, the fascia can stick together, harden, or thicken.

In addition to what we eat, of course, inflammation also depends on how much we eat. Not only are bones, joints, and fascia subjected to greater stress due when a person is overweight, more fat is also stored in the fatty tissue (which also belongs to fascia), resulting in an increased release of inflammatory mediators. However, a radical diet is not recommended, as testing has shown that this leads to an enormous reduction in the production of collagen, which is very important for our fascial structure.

Additionally, certain eating behaviors can also influence the diet-related filling of the barrel. Above all, the way we eat and our eating rhythm play a role here. Overeating, slouched posture while eating, eating even though we're not hungry, eating too fast, or eating when stressed all have a negative influence on our digestion and fill the barrel.

Because our gastrointestinal tract is sometimes very sensitive, in order to be able to process our food optimally, certain behaviors around eating are important because of their secondary effects. If, for example, we were to lie down right after a big meal, the intestine could not digest on the food properly (disturbed intestinal peristalsis); this also has a negative effect on our ability to breathe optimally. As we've learned before, inefficient breathing can fill our barrels, too.

Going for a short walk instead of lying down would probably be the better option for our digestion. In addition, our digestion works best when we eat regularly. Irregular eating messes up the rhythm of our body, making it more susceptible to disturbances. Repeated appetite control increases the allostatic load because the body can't predict when it will receive its next meal, and the more uncertain the future is, the more stress is created in the brain (allostatic overload).

OVERLOAD

Everybody's been there. We haven't had much time recently to do any exercise, but suddenly we're highly motivated because we set our new year's resolutions or are inspired by a new training approach. We're proud that now, finally, we're diligent again and are seeing the first results of our efforts. In this "high," we forget that our body hasn't had to deal with any kind of exercise in the past months and isn't used to it anymore. It tries to get stronger and fitter quickly to adapt to the demands that are put on it, but since we don't want to lose this great feeling of success and pride in our progress, we take it to the extreme compared to what the body has been used to in the past months. There might've been small warning signs already like recurrent muscle soreness or tightness and greater fatigue, but while being in a "high," we don't like to listen to them and would rather keep on pushing. Neglecting all the signs climaxes in an injury or pain coming "out of nowhere."

What most people forget is that we don't get better or stronger from training but from the recovery phase after training. If that isn't long enough or the quality of rest isn't good because we're stressed the whole time and eat unhealthy, we overload our system, and its only way out is either breaking or first sending stronger pain signals into our conscious mind to get our body to take it easy again. So in order to not overload our system, we must learn to look at the body from a rational perspective and understand that it needs its time to adapt to the load that's placed on it.

This doesn't only count for the time or repetitions, but also the magnitude of the load we're placing on the body. Even though we want the body to be exposed to load so it gets more resilient, the dose makes the poison. If the increase in load is too great too quickly, the body might not be able to deal with it anymore. Even something as mellow as stretching can become an overload for the structures if they're not yet ready for it and the stretches aren't chosen properly or executed correctly.

The body can adapt greatly to almost everything, but it needs time and gradually increased exposure instead of a "the more the better" or "the faster the better" approach we so often see. So, when we haven't worked out in a long time, we can't expect to be back to our old form right away. When pain arises after an activity, that doesn't necessarily mean we're getting old, but that the body might just not be used to it yet. It's like with drinking. If we haven't had any alcohol in the last three years, two beers will probably get us pretty drunk. Not because we aged so much and an older body just can't stand so much alcohol anymore, but rather because we haven't been drinking in a while, and our body isn't used to it anymore. This example, of course, isn't meant to inspire you to start drinking alcohol more regularly because, as we know, this will fill your barrel rather than emptying it (especially in the long run).

2.3 PSYCHO-EMOTIONAL FACTORS

When we look at the barrel metaphor, it reveals that chronic back pain is also always subject to psychological factors. However, this doesn't mean that we have to run directly to the psychologist with every little tension in the back, but merely that factors such as stress, anxiety, and worry can always be used to explain the pain as well. Recent scientific findings about how stress affects the microbiome in our gut and how the microbiome on the other hand affects our brain prove that the close relationship between body and mind exists. And yet many people still prefer to rely solely on biomedical diagnoses.

Furthermore, my experience in recent years taught me that the mind–body connection does exist. I heard so many back-pain sufferers say that stress is always contributing to their pain, and they mostly feel their backs when they're highly stressed by something.

In any case, working on the psychological factors can significantly increase the body's ability to cope with occurring disorders. If we also strengthen ourselves psychologically, this can certainly lead to a reduction of symptoms or even complete recovery.

2.3.1 AN UNFAVORABLE ATTITUDE TOWARD PAIN

You're in pain? One thing's for sure, your body is functioning great because pain is simply one of many feedback mechanisms the body has to bring imbalances to our attention. Just like that thirsty feeling we get when receptors in the blood register that the salt concentration is too high or the blood volume too low. The body sends signals to the brain that urge us to drink in order to bring those concentrations back into balance.

However, when you're having a stressful day, you might miss your body's signals and forget to drink. The same goes for pain. When you're stressed, you might miss those other signals your body is sending out that could've prevented your pain—for example, changing your posture after sitting in a slouched position for too long. Your conscious mind needs to decide what's more important: getting all the work done that's on your desk, or changing your posture occasionally in order to not strain your muscles. Your psychology and how you perceive your environment play an important role when it comes to pain.

Nonetheless, for a long time, scientists were convinced that they could explain pain with a simple mechanical model as follows: You bump your chin against something; the signal goes up to the brain; and a sensation of pain is triggered. Today, however, we know from pain research that the entire pain-triggering process is much more complex. If a danger is perceived in the affected tissue through the nociceptors, these send a signal via the spinal cord to the brain. Yet, this does not simply process the incoming signals and automatically release pain-inducing substances. Instead, a complex analysis and interpretation of this stimulus takes place in a fraction of a second, with the brain having to consider a wide variety of additional information.

This information includes:

- danger evaluation,
- belief systems,
- past similar situations,
- future expectations, and
- other more urgent dangers.

Only after this analysis when the brain considers the pain trigger to be more meaningful than, for example, moving the arm, producing sweat, or speaking, does it send out certain chemicals that make us feel pain. So, it's important to understand that pain is actually not a bad thing. It merely makes us aware of the danger. You can imagine it's like a fire alarm that signals us to get to safety.

Sometimes this warning system can fail. Some children, for example, grow up without any feeling of pain and often injure themselves seriously because their bodies can't anticipate the danger. Their lives are filled with lots of restrictions, and life expectancy isn't as high as it is for people with normal-functioning pain systems. On the other hand, people with a missing body part often experience what is known as "phantom pain" in the missing limb.

However, the system can also simply overreact and even cause pain during normal movement. This happens when the nociceptors have become too sensitive and send out pain signals even at the slightest stimulus. This would be like our fire alarm sounded when only a small candle was burning. The experts call this effect "peripheral sensitization," or, if the central nervous system is affected, "central sensitization." In this case, we could say that our barrel shrinks and immediately overflows even though there are significantly less biopsychosocial factors. The intensity of our pain also depends on how sensitive the pain receptors are, showing that the sensation of pain is an extremely individual thing and that injury or damage to our body isn't the same as pain.

Note that this individual pain threshold can be influenced. When the brain receives a pain signal from the body via chemical substances, it sends either pain-relieving or pain-enhancing signals to the respective spot. If we step into a pin, it hurts. Meanwhile, if we run away from a lion, we won't even know it. In such a dire and dangerous situation, the pain is reduced by the brain releasing substances such as norepinephrine, serotonin, or endorphins. This process is called **descending inhibition**.

However, the brain doesn't always need a dangerous situation for this. We can also activate this mechanism by doing things that give us joy, have lots of meaning for us, or that foster loving relationships with other people. Even our favorite music and pleasant smells can help reduce pain.

On the other hand, there's the **descending facilitation**. Our body now sends substances to the affected area, making the tissue even more sensitive. The more sensitive it is, the more likely it is to hurt. This mechanism can mean that an old injury still hurts even though it's long been healed. It's activated when we anticipate the pain because we think it should hurt because we've heard things like: "There's now bone on bone in your joint" or "You have the spine of an 80-year-old!" Often it's also overprotective relatives or friends who unintentionally make us even more afraid by persuading us that we must take care of ourselves and take special care not to do anything wrong.

Recent studies confirm that the more attention we pay to the damage and the more we regard it as something bad, the more the descending facilitation works, and the stronger and longer the pain is. Typical things a back-pain patient says as a result are: "Something dangerous is happening in my body!" "The pain will stop me from being able to do the things that are most important to me." "I'll probably be disabled like my colleague who had the same issue."

What happens to these patients as a result s is that they begin to move very carefully because they think something is damaged in their back (remember that in 90% of the cases nothing really bad in the spin can be found) and could become even worse. This fear-avoidance behavior then leads to tension, far too little movement, and even more compression on the intervertebral discs due to the constant protective behavior.

In section 2.1, we learned that at least 30% of all people with herniated discs don't even know that they have those issues because there were never any symptoms. These people were spared in their favor from the descending facilitation, which can be quickly set in motion by a diagnosis such as a herniated disc.

It's important to understand these mechanisms because then we no longer think it's the physical damage alone that causes pain, and we must be extremely careful with our backs. Rather, we know that even though all pain is fundamentally real, no matter how it's triggered, we can do a lot to alleviate it by emptying our barrel or at least by stopping descending facilitation to prevent it from shrinking.

I believed for years what my doctor had told me at the time, that I had better be careful and not play sports so much anymore because without the cartilage and outer meniscus, the bone rubs against bone, and if I continued to strain my knee, I'd need an artificial knee joint in a few years.

I believed what my doctor said for almost a decade, and every time I felt a little more pain in my knee after playing soccer, I was afraid that my doctor's prediction would now come true. So, I reduced my playing amount, and, if at all, only did sports with low knee loads. As a result, the pain level stayed pretty low, but remained permanently until I researched pain and learned that it wasn't only the structures that caused me lasting pain, but also my beliefs. I then gave myself permission to believe that I could become completely pain free and could play soccer again at some point. That's why I stopped always checking in with my knee because doing so meant I was basically anticipating the pain to increase again. For example, after jogging, I told myself instead that I won't let the pain stop me because my knee is strong enough.

It was clear to me that after such a long time, without any greater challenges, the structures would at first be somewhat irritated. But that doesn't mean bone rubs on bone because that would actually be way more painful.

After gradually increasing the intensity of my training and doing additional exercises to improve my muscular and functional deficits, I was able to start playing soccer again, and the condition of my knee improved from time to time.

We have now widely accepted that there's a **placebo effect**. That means that there can be a cure if we think we're being cured, even though there was no active ingredient in the drug. What few people know, however, is that there's also a **nocebo effect**. According to this, pain can also get worse if we believe, for example, that we should have severe pain because of the damage. Even though it's not easy to take advantage of the placebo effect, we want to try doing as much as possible to prevent the impact of the nocebo effect.

This doesn't mean that we should trivialize the pain and not take it seriously, or even think that we have to endure it. On the contrary, it's clear that there is a problem that can continue to fill the barrel, but we don't freak out, because we know that our body can handle it very well if we just focus on emptying the barrel and changing our beliefs and expectations.

So, I hope that if you have chronic or periodic pain yourself that you, too, will stop believing that your body is extremely fragile, worn, or weak. I want to inspire you to believe that your pain can disappear despite the wear and tear. If you have periodic or chronic pain, you will probably know that there are days when your back is less painful and then days when the pain is much worse for no apparent reason.

Do you think on these "bad" days the wear and tear is more? Or maybe it depends more on various biopsychosocial factors, so that on these days maybe only your barrel is full, or your catastrophizing thoughts have shrunk it?

Pain is always a feedback, either to change something on the outside (load) or on the inside (attitude). Whichever way we choose, it always starts with not seeing ourselves as victims of our circumstances because then we will not change anything at all.

Rather, we should internalize that we are not worse off because our body is already so "worn out," but instead feel blessed because we have such a resilient body, which, despite enormous strain and signs of wear and tear, can still function perfectly and bring us joy and better quality of life if we give it the chance to do so.

2.3.2 NEGATIVE STRESS

Negative stress (distress) is always one of the causes of back problems as well as many other diseases and can fill the barrel rapidly. It can have the most diverse causes and characteristics.

The term "stress" originally comes from material testing and means tension, distortion, or bending. While this was referring to only physical stress, psychological stress is the one that most people complain about in this day and age. Psychological stress can be defined as "...a biochemical process that only takes place in the head and is caused by the fear of not being able to get something done. Stress is not caused by someone else, but only by the stressed person himself" (Becker, 1990). This means that the way in which stress affects the human organism depends on our perception of the stressor, thus triggering either distress or eustress (positive stress) in us.

Distress can be caused by outer or inner conflicts, difficult challenges, worry, meaninglessness, fears, and anxiety. A difficult challenge, especially in an area that's very important for us, activates a defense plan through which we call on the fight, flight, or freeze responses. This is deeply rooted in our evolutionary history and ensures that the release of cortisol and adrenaline increases our blood pressure and heartbeat, our attention, and our muscle reactions (sympathetic activation), while the functions that are not immediately needed, such as digestion, reproduction, or immune defense (parasympathetic activation), are inhibited.

For a short time, as with stress breathing, this is not a problem for us. However, if this state becomes a permanent condition, it can be accompanied by anxiety, worry, or depression and can lead to exhaustion, loss of performance, and physical tension. How much time we need to adapt to the stressor becomes more crucial than whether the stressor occurs again and again. If we had a major cataclysmic event, and we kept on suffering for months or years, this would add to our distress levels. But if we're able to adapt and move on with our life quicker, the influence of that stressor isn't as great. So, we often like to blame our back problems on all the distress we experience, but in the end, it also depends on us and our attitude toward the stressor whether and to what extent we experience distress.

On the other hand, there is positive eustress, which has a positive influence on the physical and mental functioning of the organism. In fact, we absolutely need this kind of stress because it enables us to become more efficient and evolve. Eustress arises when we do things that give us joy or are meaningful to us. At the end of a really busy day, if we accomplished meaningful tasks and achieved our goals, we don't feel completely worn out and distressed, but rather we feel fulfilled. That leads to a secretion of hormones which can very well empty our barrel. Unfortunately, not many people are able to preserve this kind of stress for the long run, and most people nowadays are more exposed to distress and its negative health consequences.

Another definition of stress is "the inability to adapt to a changing environment." In our modern, technological times, being able to adapt to the rapid changes is probably more important than ever before. When someone resists using new technology like computers, smartphones, or self-driving cars, they eventually won't be able to get along well in everyday life, and they create obstacles that might cause them a lot of distress. From a health perspective, adapting to things we just can't change or developments we can't stop is crucial for our mental health as it lowers our stress levels.

2.4 SOCIAL AND ENVIRONMENTAL FACTORS

We live in a society in which we are daily exchanging with other people, even if only over social media. Interacting with people from different cultural backgrounds is higher than ever before. At the same time, since we're living in an environment shaped by industrialization and technological progress, we face unprecedented challenges and an incredible flood of information that our brains must process at lightning speed. Due to the inexorable, rapid changes in our socio-ecological living conditions, a high degree of adaptability is particularly important to prevent our barrel from being filled too much by distress based on social and environmental factors.

The social factors are directly related to the psychological ones, since in the end it's always our mental condition that determines how we perceive and interpret interactions with other people. Sometimes a social pain trigger, such as the rejection from others or exclusion from a group, can be felt in immediate physical pain, which also shows the close relationship to the physical-biological level.

2.4.1 MISSING SOCIAL SUPPORT

Our social life has a greater influence on our health than we might think. Because interactions with others are also always based on our perceptions of the situation, it can either stress us negatively and fill our barrel or support us and help us empty the barrel. If we feel uncomfortable in the presence of certain people and wish to get out of the situations but we can't, it can fill up the barrel, whereas loving, supportive, and happy relationships with our friends can empty the barrel. So if kids are sitting in front of their smartphones to talk to their friends on Facebook, Zoom, or Instagram, it might not only be harmful to their health because the social exchange also helps them to empty their barrel.

While supportive, caring social contacts are especially important when we have acute pain because they enable us to manage everyday tasks, when it comes to chronic pain, overly careful social support can induce further catastrophic thinking in ourselves. As we learned in the previous section about our attitudes toward pain, this will fill the barrel even more and lead to greater pain. Therefore, the support we get from others shouldn't be too worried or fearful.

While it might be helpful to meet other people who suffer from pain as well in order to learn from their stories, focusing too much on the pain and worst-case scenarios in conversations with them might not be the best strategy to reduce pain in the long run.

On the other hand, the famous "Cyberball" study showed that feeling socially isolated has negative effects on our health. In this study, the test person was rejected by others and couldn't participate in an online game called Cyberball. The result was significant social pain represented similarly in the brain as physical pain and that lead to the excretion of inflammatory chemicals. Social isolation is therefore recognized as a significant risk factor for diseases similar to the effects of smoking.

While those incidents of rejection lead to those acute effects in most people, being alone can also be enjoyable for people who are used to a lot of social stress. As mentioned before, attitude toward stress depends very much on the situation the person is in and their perception of it.

In addition, we often adapt to the behavior of our fellow human beings. Our mirror neurons are responsible for this. When we observe behavior patterns in other people, these nerve cells ensure that we automatically want to perform the same action ourselves. While the mirror neurons help us walk in other people's shoes and encourage our empathy, they can also tempt us to copy the unhealthy behavior of others.

If, for example, we have colleagues who aren't interested in health at all and bring unhealthy snacks to work every day, it's more difficult to resist the temptation and change our own behavior to more healthy eating habits.

Of course, we cannot expect to have only supportive and loving relationships because life always brings its challenges. But we can often choose the people we surround ourselves with or actively demand support of them if certain things are particularly important to us.

2.4.2 UNHEALTHY ENVIRONMENTAL INFLUENCES

Our back health is not only influenced by our social relationships, but also by our environment. This includes, in particular, our workplace, schools, and our home.

If a therapist or trainer isn't able (or simply doesn't have the time) to really empathize with the client and their life and doesn't address their living conditions before demanding behavioral changes, long-term failure is often inevitable. Simply telling the client what they're doing wrong without addressing individual circumstances can lead to frustration and blame.

If we sit for hours and hours every day at a desk that doesn't meet ergonomic standards or if we have to perform repetitive, straining movements all day long, our path to sustainable back health becomes enormously difficult. Moreover, if we're exposed to increased radiation in our home, if we're disturbed at night by too much light or noise, or if we don't have a mattress that adapts to our spinal form, then we cannot even recover properly at night. Relaxing sleep is indispensable for our health.

If we sleep badly or too little, our body cannot regenerate optimally. Not only does this have negative effects on our mood and makes us more susceptible to stress everyday life, it also overflows our barrel.

Unpleasant smells in our environment are other, though probably less well-known, negative influences. Unpleasant smells can cause us to stop breathing normally and instead start breathing more shallowly.

So, it's not always just the lack of will to lead a healthier lifestyle, but it can also be the environment that prevents change or makes it difficult to change.

3 YOUR EFFORTLESS WAY TO BACK HEALTH

Because back problems are so complex, naturally the methods for solving them are countless and exist on all three levels of the biopsychosocial model. In this chapter we will examine a number of action steps which will help drain the barrel. These steps are part of my EFFORTLESS method, and we will use this method to find which steps work best for you.

3.1 THE EFFORTLESS METHOD

In the first two chapters of this book, we gained insight into the extensive biopsychosocial causes of back problems, learning that back problems aren't only of physical–biological nature, but also have psychosocial causes. As a result, a holistic approach is the most promising.

Although most people in our western world are subject to a lot of physical wear and tear and compensation, those can only be seen as the "matches" that will only ignite a fire when there are many psychosocial factors or strong physical strains, resulting in pain. In addition, our attitude toward the "match," or rather, the pain, also determines how strongly we feel the pain. If we have catastrophic thoughts, this increases our sensitivity to pain; when we're more relaxed about the problems, the pain can be alleviated.

In this chapter, we will look at several action steps in each area of the bio-psycho-social model that can help you empty your barrel to achieve sustainable back health and better quality of life.

Because all areas interact with each other, an improvement in one area will also bring about an improvement in another. That is why, when using my EFFORTLESS method, you can select from the 10 steps only those steps that suit you best.

When it comes to choosing the right methods for your back-health plan, no one area is preferred. Every activity has the potential to empty your barrel to such an extent that possible complaints disappear, and your quality of life is increased. We will concentrate on filtering out your own optimal action steps in order to increase the probability of your success.

When I talk to people who have back problems, I hear the same statements over and over again: "I know, I know. I should be doing something for my back." "My doctor also told me, I have to do more exercise." "I wanted to start with the back exercises, but..." It seems that the biggest problem often isn't that we don't know what we could do to help ourselves, but that we still don't do it.

On the one hand, this is simply due to other priorities. We're too busy with our jobs, with our children, with our partner, and so on, so that there's no more time to take care of our own back. The other reason is that we simply don't like the activity imposed on us, and after a long, exhausting day of work, we prefer to surrender to the numerous entertainment options instead of doing exercises for our back. We will then no longer be willing or able to put any further effort into actively working on our back health. The misconception, however, is that actions always come with effort. We usually accept the effort of an activity when something important is involved or when we have fun doing a particular activity. If something is an effort for us, then it is, by definition, difficult, tiring, or boring to do. These tasks that require more effort are often associated with difficulty and strain as well as time-consuming work.

Since we tell ourselves that we "have to" or we "should" do it, it becomes an extra burden on which we don't want to spend any more time and most likely won't, at least not in the long run. Physical training, for example, can be stressful and annoying for some people, and they often must force themselves to do it, whereas for others training is so inspiring and effortless that they can't imagine a life without it.

So, if we find something for which we might say, "I would love to do that," "that would certainly help me," or "to change that isn't a problem for me at all," then it becomes effortless because we no longer perceive it as something difficult and laborious. It also doesn't "consume" our time because we gladly accept the work involved.

When it comes to effortless activities, it doesn't necessarily mean they don't entail any kind of work. Rather, it's a matter of selecting those attempts that aren't associated with great difficulties and won't burden you more, which would actually fill your barrel even more.

With the help of my ***EFFORTLESS** method*, together we will develop a plan for sustainable back health, better quality of life, and higher performance that you can implement effortlessly.

EFFORTLESS Method

Exercises

Favorite activity

Fuel

Optimizing environment

Reason determination

Treatments

Load management

Ergonomics

Stress management

Social support

For your back-health plan, you will use only those areas that you say you can effortlessly implement. For this purpose, we will evaluate the individual areas on the *EFFORTLESS scale* (to be explained in more detail in the following section).

We will then incorporate the steps of your highest rated area into your back-health plan. The goal is to select the three areas you've given the highest EFFORTLESS values. However, you can decide for yourself whether you want to start with just one area first and then possibly add a second or third area later. It's important that you do not under- or overload yourself, but try to assess you and your life as much as possible.

We don't have to optimize all 10 areas and do everything "perfectly." Our body can tolerate a lot of unhealthy circumstances in the most unbelievable way, and it even needs these challenges to become stronger and more resilient. Therefore, small, effortless changes can often be enough to empty the barrel and spur you on. So it's important to take a well-thought-out approach to your back-health plan because the more realistic your plan is, the fewer obstacles you will encounter, and the more likely it is that your approach will be a success.

There are 10 different areas, and each one can help you if you really implement the actions purposefully. However, if you approach it half-heartedly and thoughtlessly and hope that this would be enough for you to feel a permanent change, it's likely you won't experience the desired outcome.

But we want to achieve lasting back health, and to make that happen, we have to stick with our plan. If you're fully convinced the path you chose is right, and it doesn't take too much effort to implement it, then you will experience results. If you follow your plan one step at a time, it will build momentum and soon you will have emptied your barrel sufficiently so that you do not feel pain anymore. Effortless doesn't necessarily mean that the changes won't be challenging, however. The point is that you choose the path that suits you best which means you are more likely to persevere. Brian Tracy, the world renown thought leader in personal and professional growth, says, "Every minute you spend on planning, saves 10 minutes in execution." So, let's make your time investment the most efficient and prepare your back-health plan thoroughly.

3.2 THE EFFORTLESS SCORE

Using the EFFORTLESS score, we will filter out the most promising areas for your back-health plan. How many times have we started with a high level of motivation only to realize after a few days or weeks that we've let it slip until we've given up completely and then feel bad about ourselves? Be it a new diet, fitness plan, yoga class, or the New Year resolutions, it's hard to keep motivated.

To stay motivated to keep on track with your back-health plan, we really only want to use only those action steps that are simple to implement, making it easy to stick with your plan.

What you will need to do is answer the following three questions after reading about each of the 10 areas of the method and assign them a number on a scale of 1-10 (1 = very little, 10 = a lot).

1. Conviction:

How convinced are you that the action steps in this area will help you?

Do you believe what you've read, and does it make sense that the actions can help you? Or do you think it's nonsense, unimportant, and ineffective? Or maybe you remember that similar steps have helped you in the past. It's really about what you believe, not what you hear from others. So, before just picking a high number, ask yourself: Do you believe these steps will help, or are you just thinking they could help because you heard from others that they should?

Here it's also important to consider what you think mostly fills your barrel. Is it physical-biological, psychological-emotional, or social-environmental factors? Whichever area you feel has the most influence on filling your barrel could also have the greatest influence on emptying your barrel if you resolve those factors. On the other hand, if you're already doing well in an area and see no problems there at all, the action steps won't help you much anymore. If, for example, your diet is already very anti-inflammatory, changes here probably won't have that much of an impact as the individualized exercises, if you previously were more of a couch potato. So, consider your attitude toward the exercises as well as your initial situation. Last but not least, it can sometimes help to try out new steps before saying we're convinced it will help us. So, if there's anything that sounds interesting, but you aren't sure what it will be like to execute it, just give it a try first and pick the number for your conviction afterwards.

2. Inspiration:

How much do the activities inspire you, and would you be keen on doing them?

Do you like the action steps in that area? Would you even look forward to doing them? Do you feel an inner motivation because they would mean a lot to you? Going after things that inspire you is the opposite of doing things that you think you "have" to do because somebody told you so. If an action really inspires you, you won't need much external motivation and won't expect any external reward for it. Even if the activity is a challenge for you, you want to take on that challenge because it really inspires you and gives you meaning.

3. Probability of implementation:

How likely do you think it is that you will implement the exercises?

You know yourself and your life best. Have you perhaps already started something similar before and haven't finished it? Or do you think you'd have no problem implementing and even sticking to these actions? Think about your everyday life. Do you see ways in which you can integrate the activities into your daily routine? Or are they too time consuming for you? Do you feel your life is currently too stressful to invest any time into them? Also think about your resources. Do you actually have everything you need to do those action steps? Money, time, people, space, knowledge?

The more accurately you answer these questions, the more likely the action steps will help you, and the more likely you are to stick to your back-health plan. So try to assess yourself accurately and think carefully about the particular questions. In addition, I'll give you an appraisal for each to determine whether those action steps would be relevant in your case. This can help you to better answer the question about your conviction, but should not overrule your own opinion.

Then you calculate your EFFORTLESS score for the respective area by adding up all numbers of the three questions. To create your individual back-health plan, you'll select the areas with the highest scores.

3.3 THE 10 AREAS OF THE EFFORTLESS METHOD

E F F O R T L E S S

3.3.1 EXERCISES

Exercises for a sustainable, healthy back make up the core of this book. A targeted exercise plan based on the individual, functional movement deficits is the best way to remove the compensation-related "match" and eliminate the basis for igniting a lasting fire. Therefore, this area is the most detailed. You will first learn about all the different parts of your exercise plan to get an idea of the effects of the specific exercise and understand why doing a self-test beforehand is so important.

THE FUNCTIONAL TRAINING APPROACH

Functional training is all about training the body in the way its muscle chains actually function by using three-dimensional movements. In recent years, the study of anatomy has undergone a revolution, as we've come to understand that muscles can no longer be viewed in isolation; their functions are determined by the direction of pull from their origin to their insertion alone. Our body's functions can vary depending on its position and the influence of gravity. Moreover, our muscles always function in conjunction with other muscles and the fascia that surrounds them.

Instead of strengthening only one muscle group in isolation, functional training strengthens muscle chains by performing whole-body movements. The aim is to learn efficient patterns of movement without excessive compensatory movements. This not only removes the "match" and our susceptibility to overloading, but it also lets us become more efficient in certain everyday movements.

In our modern, everyday life, we only use a fraction of the degrees of freedom that our joints actually have. As a result, true to the motto "use it or lose it," these unused joint functions are slowly but surely lost.

Functional also means preserving important motor functions into old age. While mobility restrictions may not yet play a major role for an office worker, they can become a burden later in life when it comes to getting dressed or getting up without assistance.

If we don't use our freedom of movement regularly, we can watch it disappear. In addition, we load our joints off balance, which leads to faster wear. Although this doesn't automatically mean that pain will occur, it does provide more matches for igniting a fire.

The functional training approach restores mobility to the most important joints and then integrates it together with sufficient stability into whole-body movements. This makes our movements smoother, more coordinated, and more efficient. Due to the lower energy loss and the use of our full movement capabilities, our performance capacity increases.

INDIVIDUAL FUNCTIONAL MOVEMENT DEFICITS

Since everybody is different and has compensated in their own way over the years based on the given circumstances, individualized, functional training on the way to back health is the most effective method. Giving only general advice or recommending exercises without checking the status quo of the body can be counterproductive.

For example, it's often recommended to always stretch the hip flexor muscles when having back problems. Although it might have been found that this muscle is often shortened in back-pain patients, whether tight hip flexor muscles are the problem should always be checked so that there's no overstretching of already well-stretched muscle and fascia, which could even aggravate the back pain. Even recommendations that aim for strong back or abdominal muscles can be counterproductive without appropriate tests.

Back muscles are usually already tense and should be released especially in people with a reinforced arched back. The same applies to an already excessively strong or shortened abdominal musculature, which can often be observed in people with hunched backs. When there's too much tension in one area, it can facilitate too much laxity in other areas. When we bring more balance into the overly tense areas, we can indirectly lower the laxity in those other areas.

Functional movement tests help to identify these individual functional movement deficits as well as the causes of the overloads. American functional training experts Gray Cook and Michael Boyle have invented the "joint-by-joint" theory for selecting the right tests to determine the causes of the complaints (Cook 2011). This theory states that in a dysfunctional joint, the areas directly over or under it should always be tested for their functionality, as these are the most frequent causes for compensations in the dysfunctional joint. For the lower back, these are the thoracic spine and the hips.

I had a lot of such functional movement deficits at the time I was experiencing pain. Not only did I have an immobile hip, but I also had quite the kyphosis (rounded thoracic spine). While there certainly would have been some other deficits, targeted training to eliminate the deficits in these areas was enough to relieve my lower back sufficiently and to give me freedom from pain. In my work with hundreds of back pain sufferers, I have also spotted these areas in most of them as being the main causes of their problems. In one case, it was more the hips rather than the thoracic spine that had mobility restrictions.

Although there are certainly some cases in which the causes for compensations come additionally from the feet, knees, or even jaw or vision, these are the key areas, as they are directly adjacent to the lower back, and the compensations are more evident. The purpose of the following self-tests is to check if those key areas are in relative balance or not.

Through the subsequent training of the individual functional movement deficits, the "match" in the form of our compensations can then best be removed and also prevent the ignition of fire in the long term. With the help of simple tests, the mobility of hips and shoulders can be tested. If deficits are found here, targeted mobilization exercises in these areas help to restore sufficient mobility and reduce the probability of compensation.

LEARNING BASIC MOVEMENTS

Before starting with functional training, it's necessary to acquire two basic skills: 1) tilting the pelvis posteriorly and anteriorly (see fig. 3.1) for certain exercises, and 2) learning what your neutral spine position is (see fig. 3.2 and 3.3). The neutral spine is the position of your elastic equilibrium in which there is a balance of muscle tension on both the front and back of your upper body, and you will need to know this position in certain exercises as well as in different postures you make every day.

Due to the effects of gravity, the body can reveal completely different compensatory patterns between lying or standing. So, you should practice the neutral spine position first in a lying position and then in a standing position.

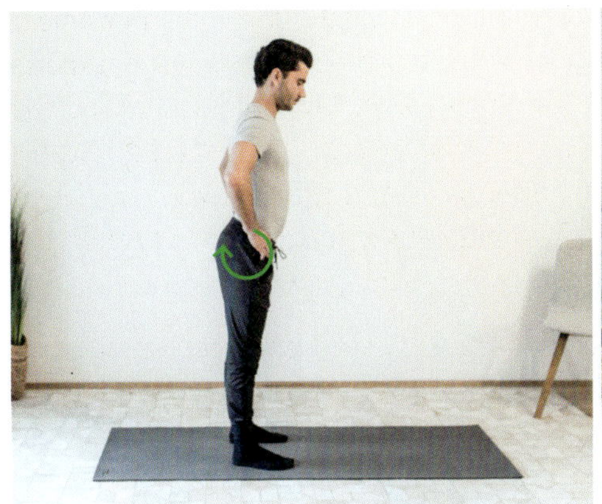
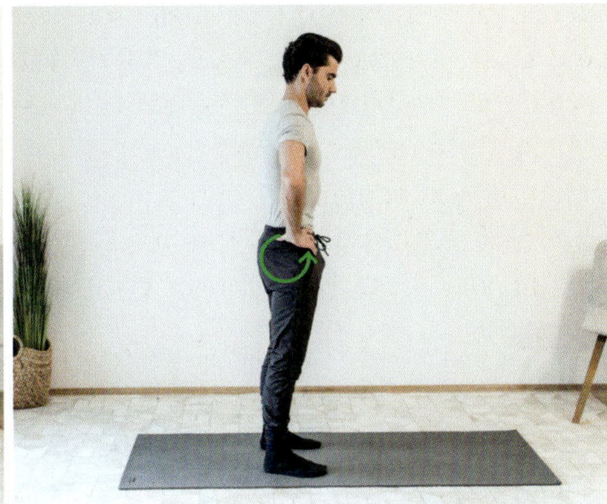

Fig. 3.1 Tilting the pelvis anteriorly and posteriorly

Stand upright, positioning your hands on the sides of your pelvis. Imagine that you have a bowl of water between your hands, resting against your pelvis. If you want to pour water out the front of the bowl, then you must tilt your pelvis forward (anterior tilt). If you want to pour water out the back of the bowl, then you must lift your pelvis (posterior tilt). Try to isolate the movement at the pelvis so that your rib cage moves as little as possible.

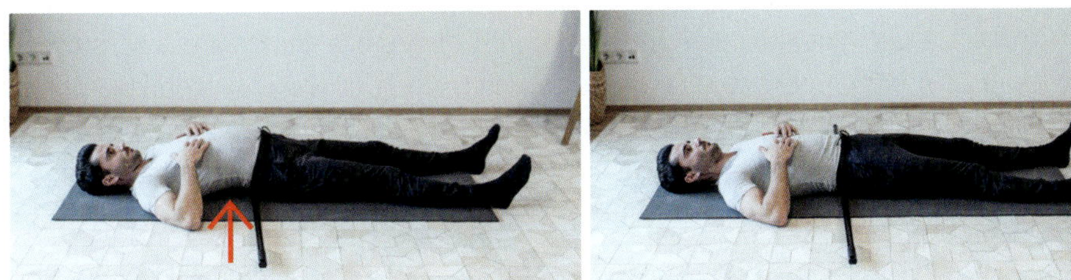

Fig. 3.2 Finding your neutral spine in a supine position

While lying flat on your back, place a bar underneath your lumbar spine, right above your pelvic crest. Lower your chin until only a fist can fit between your chin and sternum, while simultaneously stretching your neck as if someone were pushing on the back of your head. If your neck still has a high arch, put a small pillow under your head to lengthen the neck. Arch your lower back as much as possible until you feel tension in your lower back muscles. Then push your lower back down against the stick. You should feel uncomfortable pressure from the stick, but there shouldn't be any pain. The idea is to find a comfortable and aligned balance between the two extremes in which there is minimal arch in your lower back, but you don't feel any tightness in the muscles.

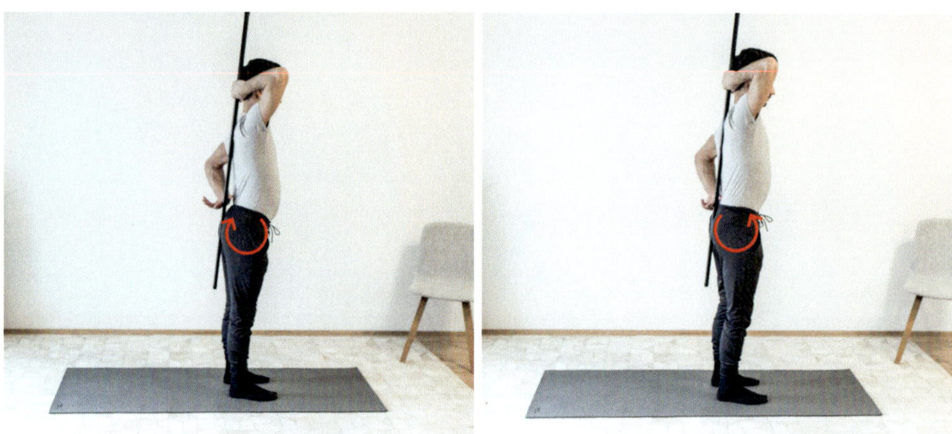

Fig. 3.3 Finding your neutral spine position in an upright position

Stand upright and hold a stick behind your back with one hand holding the bottom of the stick and one holding the top so that the stick has contact with your pelvic crest, upper back, and back of head. Position your hands so that your thumbs are between the stick and your spine. Tilt your pelvis forward, as if pouring water forward from the bowl of the pelvis, and push your rib cage forward as much as possible until you feel the space between your lower back and the stick is increasing and your lower back muscles become tight (pictured left). Then lift the pelvis up and under as much as possible so that your lower back pushes against the thumb and stick. Again, the two extreme positions are to be avoided. Find the sweet spot in between the extremes where there is minimal arch in your lower back, but you don't feel any tightness in the lower back muscles (pictured right).

TREATING FASCIA

Instead of going to get a massage, we can also self-treat our tissues. In order to loosen up fascia that is glued or matted, we can exert targeted pressure on the fascia using a massage stick and gentle, rolling and stroking movements. A simple broom stick or collapsible rod made of varnished metal works best. Similar to a sponge, the fascia will absorb liquid, which they then use to better supply nutrients while inflammation disappears. Gentle stroking is enough here, so you don't need to press deep into the tissue, as in a "trigger point" massage.

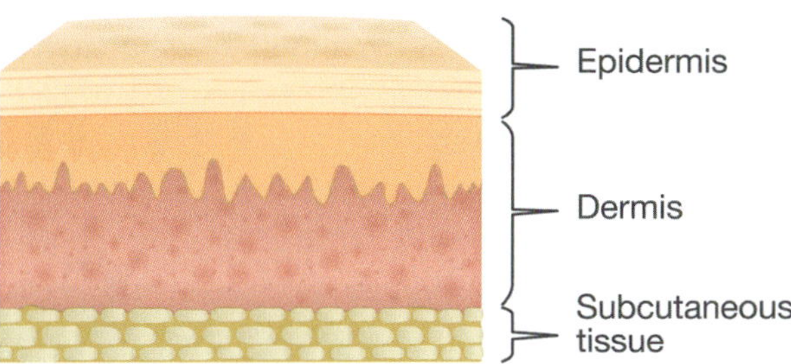

Fig. 3.4 Superficial fascia layers

If we gently stroke the skin with the stick, the adhesions of the fascial layers directly under the skin (dermis and subcutaneous tissue) are loosened; this treatment is particularly effective against tension and pain because more than 80% of the afferent nerves terminate in free nerve endings here, and most of them are responsive to mechanical tension, pressure, or shear deformation.

By treating the lower back (see fig. 3.5), the impaired awareness (proprioception) of this area that back pain sufferers often have can be improved again, and tension can be released (at least temporarily). Same counts for neck tension, which can be relieved by the treatment (see fig. 3.6).

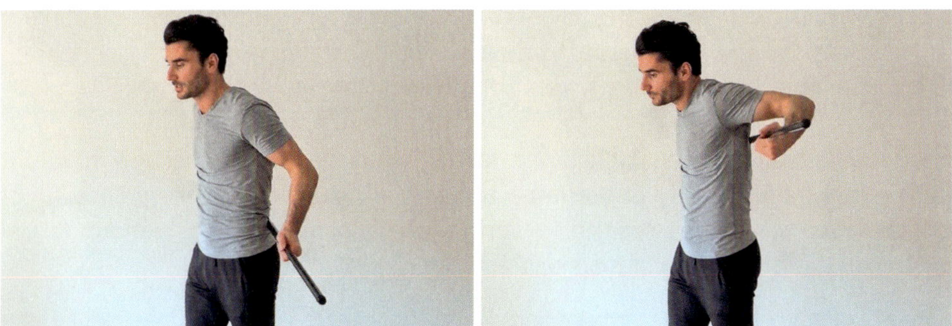

Fig. 3.5 Treating the fascia of the lower back

Standing upright, position the stick diagonally on your lower back so that it touches the big muscle next to the spine (musculus erector spinae), but not the spine itself. Apply pressure to the muscle with rapid up-and-down movements. Start with the stick above the pelvic crest and progress as high as you can. Apply more pressure to areas that feel more uncomfortable, but do so gently so that no pain occurs.

The effect is increased if the treatment is carried out directly on the skin. Apply some viscous body lotion to the respective area shortly before the treatment and work each area for at least 30 seconds. Important: Skip bones, joints, and birthmarks and stop treatment in case of sensitive skin reactions; if necessary, consult a dermatologist beforehand. Since the fascia are only treated gently, you should not feel any pain while massage the tissue, at most only a slightly unpleasant feeling.

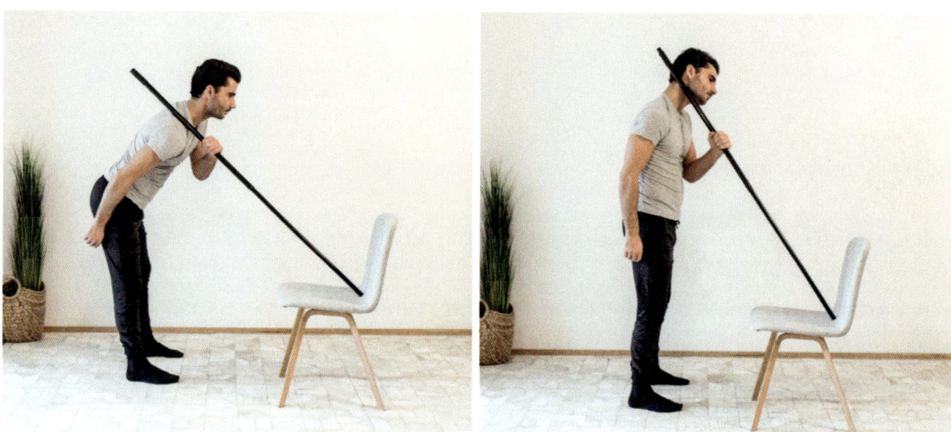

Fig. 3.6 Treating the fascia of the neck

Stand in front of a chair and press the stick at an angle against the lower part of the back of the chair. Bend forward and position the stick on your neck. Use the opposite hand to stroke your neck with small back-and-forth movements from the base at the shoulder all the way up to the ear. Pay a little more attention to areas that feel more uncomfortable, but do not apply so much pressure that you feel pain.

The increased blood flow through the fascia treatment has another advantage; it also increases the mobility of the respective area. This can reduce the probability of compensation in adjacent segments, which is why it makes sense to perform fascial treatment at the beginning of functional training.

A good example of the rapid improvement in mobility can be seen in the treatment of the feet. The treatment of the *plantar fascia* (sole of the foot) has an effect on the complete fascial backline, which spans from the big toe over the complete back of the body up to the forehead.

In order to feel the quick effects of that treatment, measure your fingertip-to-floor distance as shown in fig. 3.7 when you bend forward. Then treat your feet for one minute each (see fig. 3.8) and test the fingertip-to-floor distance again.

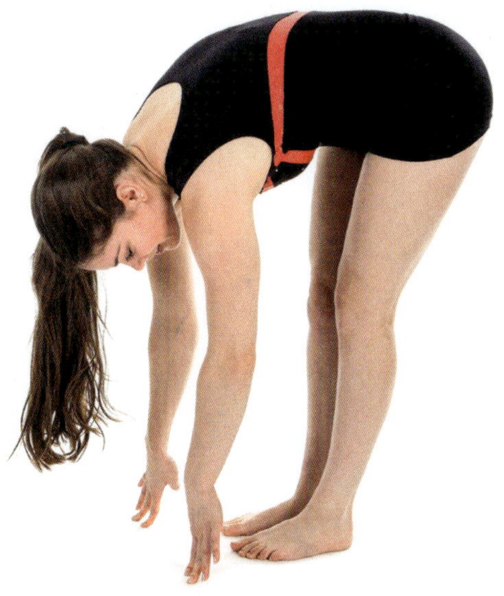

Fig. 3.7 Fingertip-to-floor test

Bend forward as far as you can while still keeping your legs completely straight. Stretch your arms toward the ground. Take note of the distance between your fingertips and the floor.

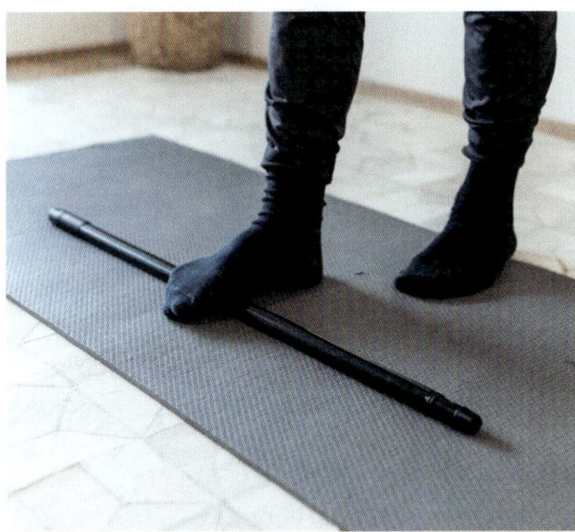

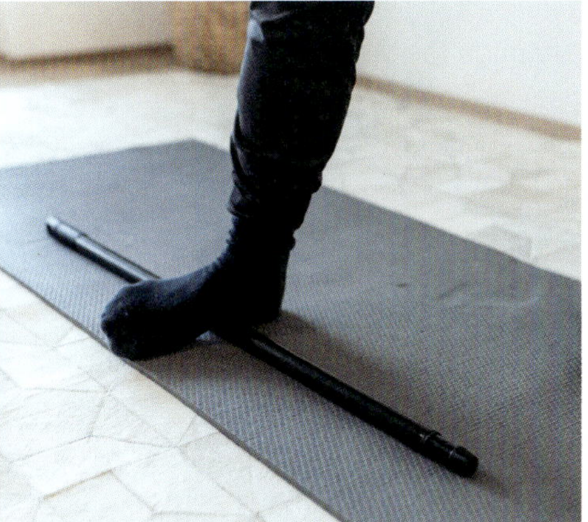

Fig. 3.8: Treating the fascia of the feet

Stand with one foot on a stick. First, roll the ball of your foot over the stick using small back-and-forth movements. Next, roll out the arch of foot by turning the knee in slightly. Roll further in areas that feel more uncomfortable, but don't apply so much pressure that there's pain. Finally, roll gently over the heel and then a few times over the entire foot. When you have completed one foot, place it down on the floor and check for increased blood circulation and a lighter feeling in the entire leg before moving on to the other foot. This exercise can also be done barefoot.

You can actually treat the fascia anywhere on the backside of your body, be it the calves, hamstrings, or lower back, and you will have the same effects on your forward bend. It's all connected.

Have you been able to narrow your finger-to-floor distance? Then the fascia exercises can help you improve your mobility. Did you get to the ground before that? Then you probably already have sufficient mobility in this fascia line. Nevertheless, your fascia can still benefit from being treated to ensure better removal of waste products and nutrient supply. In addition, fascial exercises are also able to counteract cellulite. So, I would also encourage you to try and treat the fascia of your entire body with those stroking movements. You will feel loose and relaxed afterward, and you will realize again how nice your body can feel.

Again, it's important to avoid bones, joints, and birthmarks and consult a dermatologist in case of severe skin reactions. For some areas, you have to be creative to reach those areas and to put enough pressure on the skin. Pressing the stick against a chair or the wall when treating the neck, for example, can be helpful to anchor the stick to create enough pressure.

Although the fascia, as we've learned in section 2.2.3, can be seen as an origin point for pain and tension, the causes for this are multifactorial as we already learned. While the main focus of the functional training approach is still to minimize compensations, good preparatory work can be done with these fascial treatments.

TRAINING BREATHING PATTERNS

Breathing is one of the most important functions of our body. To prevent breathing dysfunctions from filling our barrel, the targeted improvement of our breathing functionality is very important.

Our breathing is controlled by the autonomous nervous system and functions involuntarily. Although we could still influence it ourselves, automation allows us to concentrate on other things in everyday life and not on actively inhaling and exhaling. Breathing should be autonomous, rhythmic, and adapted to the situation. The breathing exercises are all goal related and will be part of your training plan. Knowing why you're doing them will empower you to use them whenever you think you need them.

But before learning about those different exercises, it's good to know your current breathing capability. A simple test that gives you a rough idea of the functionality of your breathing is the *Breath Hold Test* (see fig. 3.9).

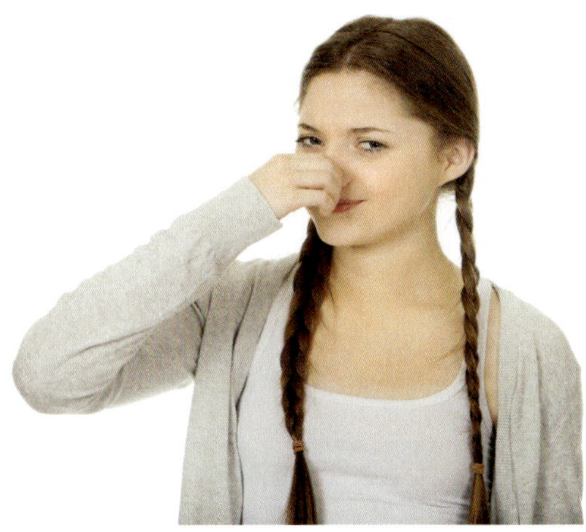

Fig. 3.9: Breath hold test

Breathe out completely through your nose and then close your nostrils with your thumb and index finger. Measure the time you can hold your breath and note the first urge to take a breath. If that point is over 20 seconds, your breathing appears to function well. Feeling an urge to breathe before holding for 20 seconds could be a sign of compensation.

Even though only a few people nowadays still manage to exceed the 20-second mark, it's important to continue to work to improve on this. One way is to simply perform this test several times a day as an exercise. You should do this five times in a row to the point where the need to catch air comes back. This won't only help to normalize your breathing, but also to clear a stuffy nose.

A common reason for a poor result in this test is that we have adopted flat breathing, whereby the body has adapted its oxygen uptake and energy supply to a pattern of quickly inhaling and exhaling without any break in between. Because of that, its perception of what's normal has changed. This gives us the feeling of having to breathe in again more quickly, which in turn further facilitates our flat breathing and permanently activates our sympathetic nervous system.

In order to change our body's "normal," we can practice extending our exhalation phase (see fig. 3.42). This makes our parasympathetic muscles more active, and by lowering the thorax, our diaphragm is positioned in such a way that it can be better activated by the subsequent inhalation. In addition, forced exhalation can activate the deep abdominal muscles that stabilize the spine and stretch the diaphragm. As a result, our body no longer has to overload the neck muscles to "suck in air," so neck tensions can also disappear.

In people with a reinforced arched back, the muscles at mid back (the lower six ribs) in particular are shortened and tense, preventing the rib cage from expanding sufficiently and the diaphragm from being positioned correctly. Therefore, mobilizing these muscles through targeted breathing into the back can help (see fig. 3.21).

On the other side, there are many people with a hunched back whose front sides are tight. Doing the front breathing exercise (see fig. 3.32) opens the front side of the body, elongates the abdominal muscles, opens the chest, and stretches the pelvic floor muscles.

The pelvic floor muscles are not only important for preventing incontinence, but they are also crucial for our spinal health as they build the foundation for our spinal stability. Plus, learning to activate them accurately can help to counteract stress-related shoulder breathing. In the pelvic floor breathing exercise (see fig. 3.65), we consciously breathe into the pelvic floor, trying to expand the pelvis when breathing in (activating muscles eccentrically) and then contracting them when breathing out.

While the aforementioned breathing exercises are each part of the upcoming training plans (which ones you use are determined by your weaknesses), there are two basic exercises that you should learn independently of your self-test outcomes.

With the first exercise, you can practice all three phases of inhalation to help you regain the normal breathing mechanism in training as well as everyday life. The balloon breathing exercise (fig. 3.10) is well suited for this purpose.

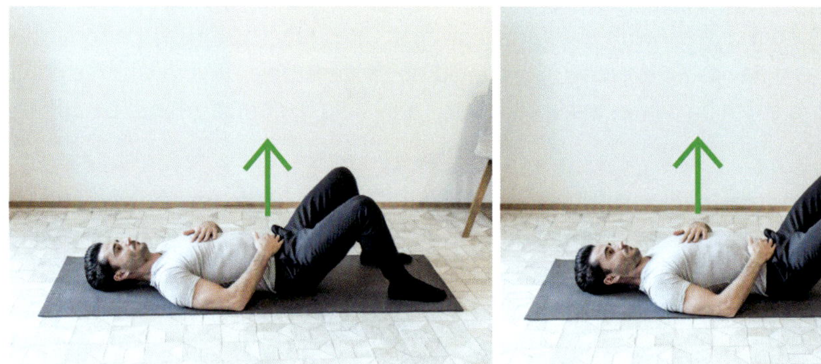

Fig. 3.10: Balloon breathing

> Lie on your back with knees bent comfortably and feet flat on the floor. Place one hand on your stomach and the other on your chest. Breathe in through your nose, bringing air into your lower abdomen, lifting your lower hand. Similar to a balloon filling with air, you will slowly fill up the rib cage with air until your upper hand also lifts. Finally, let your shoulders lift slightly to get as much air into your lungs as possible. When you breathe out through the nose, let your chest deflate first and your stomach last. Use the hands as feedback to measure the progressive inhalation and exhalation.

Expanding our chest in all directions with the three-dimensional breathing exercise (fig. 3.11) is important to ensure optimal, autonomous breathing without overstraining certain muscles. If the chest expands far enough in all directions so that the lungs can be filled with sufficient oxygen, exhalation takes place automatically at the end of the inhalation phase (as with an inflated balloon when it's released) while the diaphragm is optimally activated.

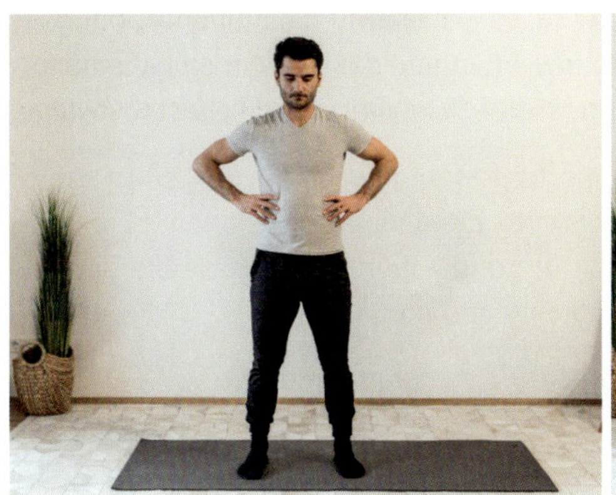
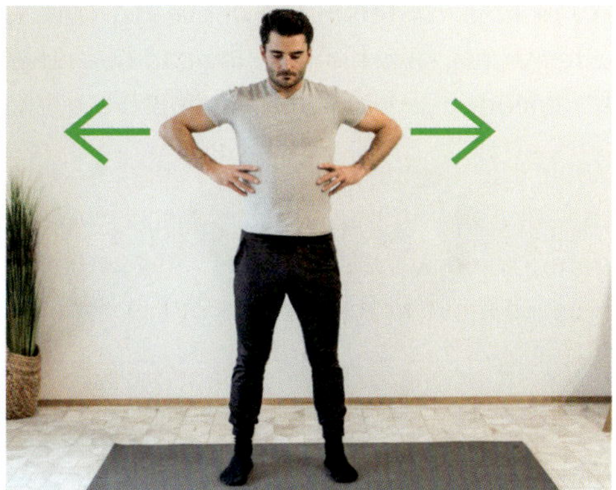

Fig. 3.11: Three-dimensional breathing

Stand up tall and position your hands on the sides of your rib cage. Breathe in as deeply as possible through your nose and expand your belly and rib cage simultaneously in all directions, meaning the ribs expand forward, out to the sides, and back so that your hands are pushed out wide. Also, push your elbows out to the side to help stop your shoulders from lifting into the ears. Then exhale completely through your nose to keep the rib cage expanded. To do this successfully, you must engage your abdominal muscles fully. With every inhalation, work to expand the rib cage more, stretching all the muscles around it while activating your core muscles. Use those same muscles to keep the expansion of the torso as you exhale.

Note that in your everyday life you still want to breathe automatically, so while it might be helpful to stop and use some of the breathing techniques every now and then, simply observing the breath without "having to change" it calms the mind and helps normalize breathing.

MOBILITY TRAINING

On the way to a sustainably healthy back, mobility helps us, above all, to not compensate so much in our everyday movements. Having sufficient mobility is the basis for free and smooth movements, but mobility is not exactly the same as flexibility.

Flexibility is usually understood as the degree of freedom of a joint. This is determined by measuring from the end of moving the joint to the end range of that specific joint. Mobility, on the other hand, describes the ability to actively move your own joints into those end ranges. The difference between mobility and flexibility is that, with flexibility, the body part is moved as far as possible with your own muscle power instead of being moved to the end range by another person or with the help of an object.

An example of this is the active leg raise (see fig. 3.17). Here the mobility is tested—in other words, how high the leg can be actively lifted (without compensatory movements). If someone else would join and push the leg up farther, flexibility would be tested instead.

While the flexibility of a joint makes an important statement about the condition of the surrounding muscles and fascia, mobility is even more meaningful when it comes to determining what movements in everyday life or during sports really look like because here we move in the degrees of freedom of mobility and not flexibility.

If we sit at the desk and want to turn to reach for the printer, no one will come and try to turn us around at the shoulder. So, the functional consideration and targeted improvement of mobility is of higher importance, while flexibility is the basic prerequisite, which, as previously shown, can also be improved by targeted fascia treatment.

STABILITY TRAINING

The basic aim of this training is to achieve a balance between mobility and stability, as this leads to optimum alignment of our joints. It's only when we have sufficient stability in addition to mobility that we can make optimum use of the degrees of freedom of our joints in our whole-body movements and do not fall, out of weakness, into more relaxed positions in which our passive structures (joints, ligaments, spine, etc.) can become overloaded. Moreover, if the brain perceives that we don't have enough stability in certain areas (e.g., inner thighs), it will go more into flexion in other areas (e.g. the spine) to secure itself, and we end up looking like someone with duck feet and a humped back (see fig. 3.12).

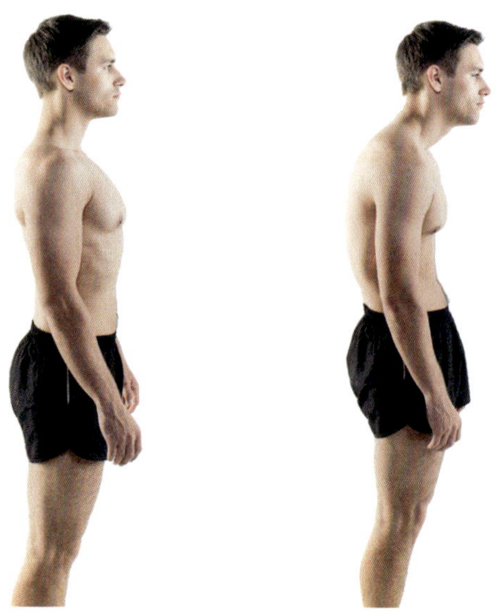

Fig. 3.12: Humpback posture; the chronically flexed upper back posture (kyphosis) has many causes. A lack of stability in certain areas of the body is one important contributor.

Stability actively keeps our body together and holds it upright against gravity. The less stable we are, the greater the risk that we will stress our passive structures. If, for example, we can no longer hold a plank position, we sag, and the main load must be carried by our spine (see fig. 3.13). Since it's been proven that the back is healthier the greater the static endurance of the core is, it's important to train that the time before we start to sag, in this plank example, is prolonged or in general that a core-challenging position can be hold longer and longer.

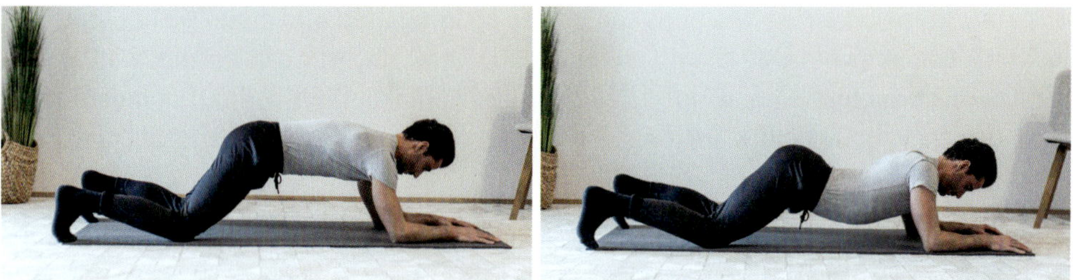

Fig. 3.13: Sagging in plank position

In this position, the spine is supposed to be kept in its neutral position. When the core muscles get tired and lose their stabilizing function, we begin to sag in the low back. This causes increased stress on the spine.

Since we don't remain in a single position all day, especially while playing sports, it's important to train dynamic stability during functional training as well. In these stability exercises (see fig. 3.14), certain segments are moved while others are kept stable. The movement must be controlled by the central nervous system in such a way that the muscles required for stabilization are activated reflexively to prevent the passive structures from being overloaded. If the muscles fire too late or not at all, there is likely a control problem or bad timing of the control.

During this exercise, as soon as the arm slides forward, the deep stabilizing muscles in the trunk are activated reflexively to prevent sagging and increased strain on the spine.

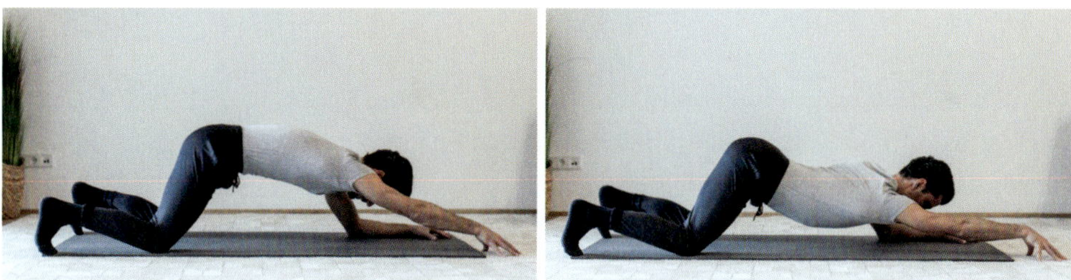

Fig. 3.14: Dynamic stability in plank position

In this exercise, the deep core muscles are supposed to be activated to stabilize the body when the arm slides forward. This should be done in a reflexive manner to prevent sagging and increased strain on the spine. When dynamic stabilization of the core isn't as strong as it should be, we sag, and the spine is more stressed.

INTEGRATING INTO "GLOBAL" EXERCISES

Compared to the more localized mobility and stability exercises which specifically target one area, those increased functions can now to be integrated into more "global" postures in which whole myofascial chains are engaged. Here, stability can ensure that we use the improved mobility in the specific body part optimally and without compensation. That way, the mobility gains are long lasting, and our everyday movements become more efficient.

A good example of a global exercise is the Hip Hinge on Stick (see fig. 3.15). Holding the arms forward creates a long lever, which means the strength endurance of the core and back muscles is trained while the calves, hamstrings, and lats are actively stretched. In addition, the targeted activation and strengthening of this chain helps to better protect the spine.

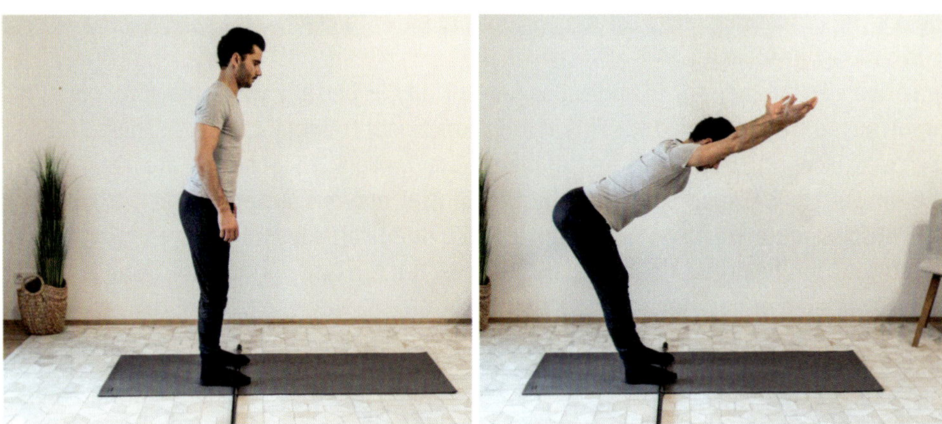

Fig. 3.15: Hip hinge on stick

Push the hips backward while standing with the balls of your feet on the stick. This activates and simultaneously stretches the complete superficial back line of our myofascial system (eccentric load). Placing the balls of your feet on the stick helps to push the hips even farther back. This helps to distribute the weight better and reduces the strain on the spine. This exercise leads to a more efficient hip hinge.

OUT-OF-ALIGNMENT MOVEMENTS

Even though the idea of having all of the joints stacked up perfectly in certain exercises is great to avoid repetitive compensatory movements and to decrease the wear and tear that comes with it, consciously moving out of that "perfect" spinal alignment comes with lots of benefits as well. As we learned previously, it helps us to train fascia and muscles the way they're supposed to work so that they don't lose function and health. That means, for example, practicing three-dimensional movements with a rounded and twisted spine or even knees that are turned inward or outward. But since we probably haven't used our body that way in a long time, it's important to start slowly and progress gradually; our nervous system needs to adapt to using its dynamic motor control in those out-of-alignment movements again.

While keeping the spine in its neutral position might be important in the beginning, for our long-term back health, we want to gradually expose our spine to out-of-alignment movements as well so we are prepared for all of the demands of everyday life or certain sports.

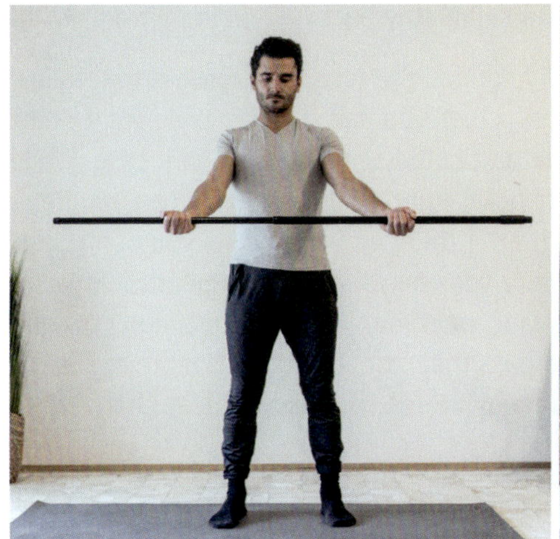

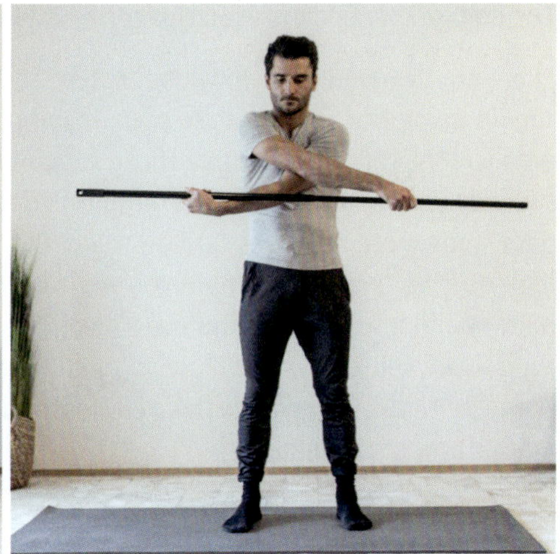

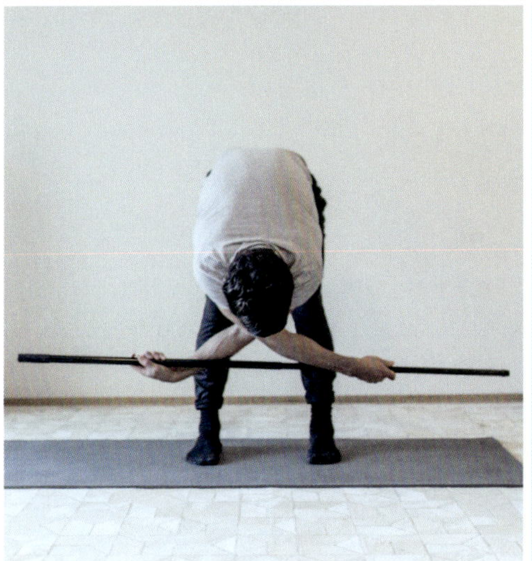

Stand with feet hip-width apart and hold a stick with arms in front of you and palms facing up. Then turn the stick so your arms are crossed over. The hands should be so far apart that you feel a stretch in your upper back. Next, pull your hands together gently, bringing your chin to your chest and bending forward as far as possible while still keeping your legs straight or only very slightly bent. Maintain this position and breathe deeply into your belly and rib cage so that you feel your back widen whenever breathing in.

Fig. 3.16: Forward fold with stick

Rounding the spine in the Forward fold with stick (fig. 3.16) is fine if our system can already bare it. If it can't and you feel pain when doing this, you have two options: either you stick with the in-alignment exercises and come back to it once you've created sufficient mobility and stability, or you still expose yourself to those out-of-alignment movements but use support to get you there. The support can be a chair, the wall, another person, and so on, just be creative. The faster your brain learns that this position isn't dangerous, the less likely it is to create pain, and eventually you can do it even without the support.

YOUR INDIVIDUALIZED TRAINING PLAN

The core of this book is exercises for a sustainably healthy back.

There are five areas which will be tested, and if you fail the test, the exercises that follow should be part of your exercise plan. If you pass a test, you can skip the exercises for that area so that you only practice those which are particularly important in your case. While this way you will get the most "bang for your bucket," of course with every test you don't pass come more exercises for you to do. But even if there are many tests you don't pass, look at it as greater potential for you to empty your barrel and bring about long-term back health and vitality. And even if you're a long way from passing a test, don't give up right away, thinking you will never be able to pass that test. The body is more malleable than you think. Doing specific exercises on a regular basis can lead to great changes, no matter how old you are.

Each area will have the following seven building blocks:

1. Self-test
2. Fascial treatment
3. Breathing exercise
4. Two mobility exercises
5. One stability/activation exercise
6. Two in-alignment exercises
7. One out-of-alignment exercise

All you need for the self-tests is a yard (meter) stick (broom stick, collapsible rod, or wooden stick), a practice mat, and some space on a wall.

Test modalities:

- Try out the exercises according to the instructions in the description and make sure you check the compensatory movements.
- Only allow two attempts to pass a test.
- If you're unsure whether you have passed the test, always choose "failed."
- If a test is not passed on one side, the whole test is considered "failed."
- If sharp pain occurs during a test, cancel the test and have a doctor examine you if necessary.

It would make sense to practice at least three times a week. If you are already advanced, you can do it five times a week for even better effects. It would be advisable to do the exercises in the morning. This has the advantage that you would benefit the entire day from a more relaxed back. If you do lots of bends and twists for the spine, a 30-minute walk before that would be important to rehydrate and decompress your discs to counteract the effects of sleep. If you do the exercises in the evening, however, they would have the advantage that you might be able to move deeper into the positions, and they could provide a more restful sleep.

Before you start training, have a look at the basics from section 3.1.4. Also bear in mind that the exercises are not meant to generate an intense burning sensation in your muscles, but to improve the functionality of your body in various movements. If you notice that you have problems with the number of repetitions or the execution of an exercise, reduce the number, skip the exercise, or try to tweak it so that it doesn't discomfort you anymore. On the other hand, you can also perform more repetitions or try to make the exercise harder if you feel very underchallenged.

1. Hip Flexion:

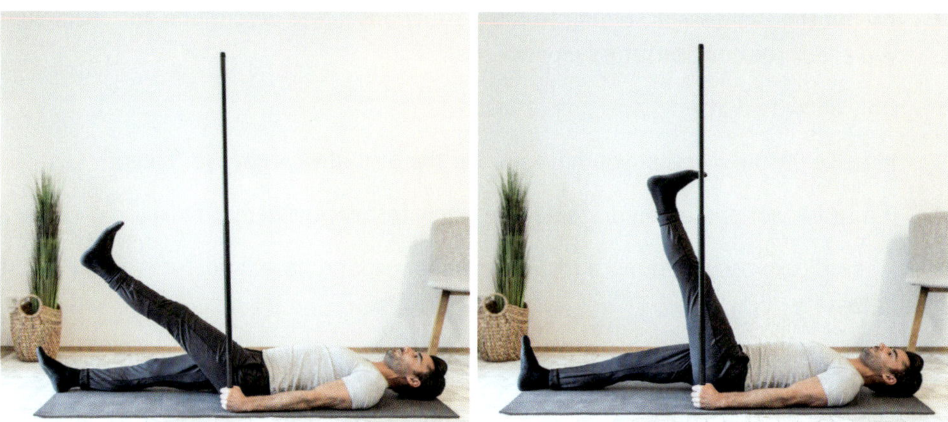

Fig. 3.17: Testing hip flexion mobility

Lie on your back. Hold the stick up perpendicular to the floor with the arm holding the stick completely stretched out next to you on the floor. Lift the leg on the same side as the stick as far as possible while keeping it completely straight and pulling the toes toward the knee. You passed this test if your toes reach the height of the stick without performing any compensatory movements. Repeat the test on the other side.

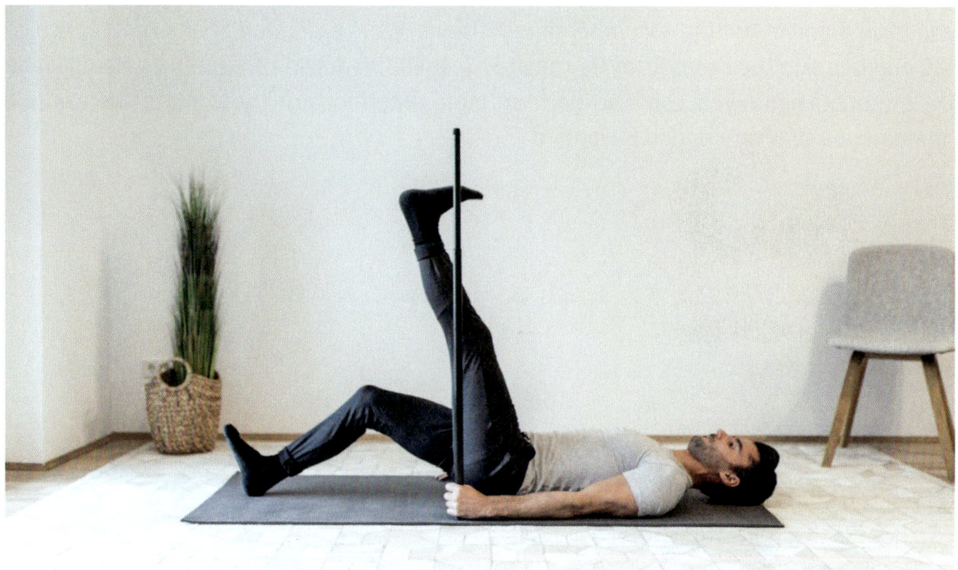

Fig. 3.18: Compensation 1: Bending the leg that is on the ground

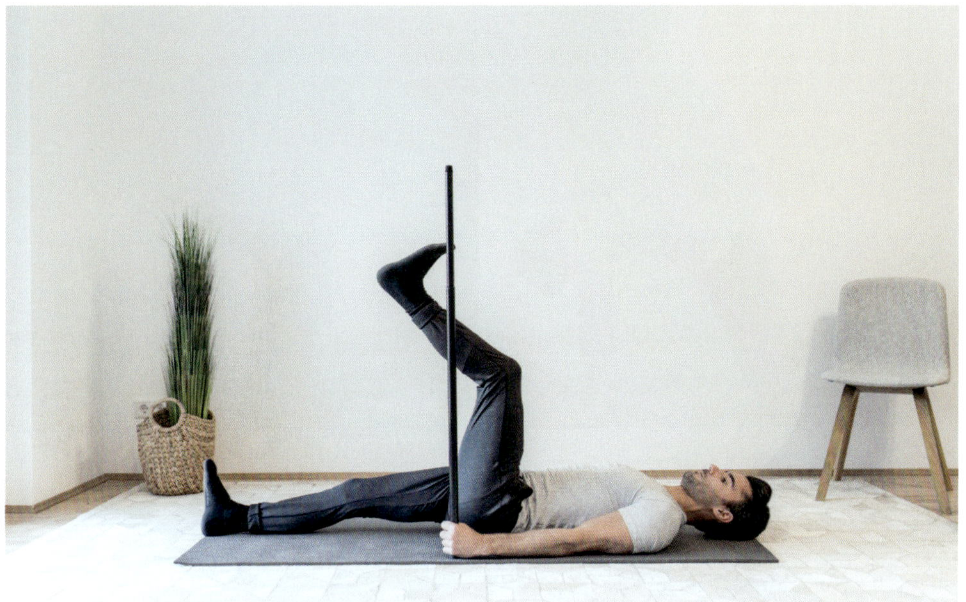

Fig. 3.19: Compensation 2: Bending the raised leg

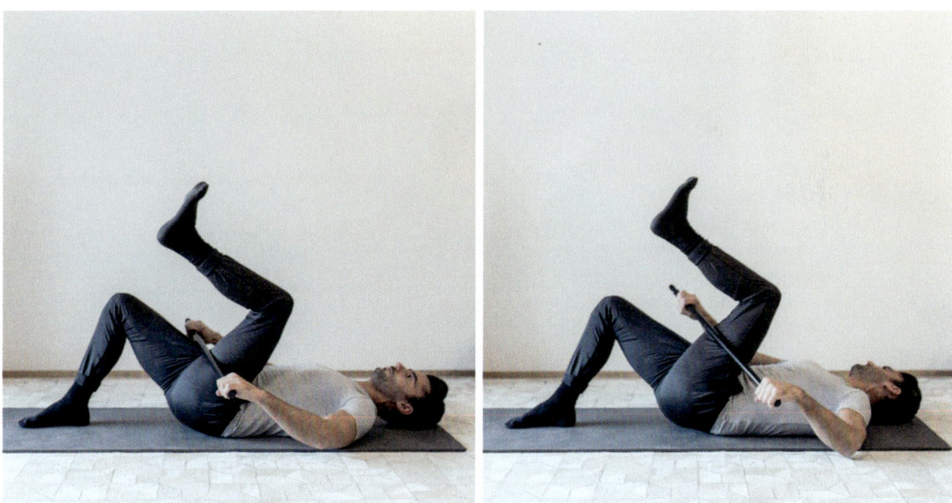

Fig. 3.20: Treating the fascia of the hamstrings (1 minute per side)

Lying on your back, lift one leg up and place the stick across the hamstrings. Then massage the hamstrings with rapid back-and-forth movements from where they attach to the pelvis up to the back of the knee. Pay a little more attention to areas that feel more uncomfortable, but do not massage so hard that you feel pain.

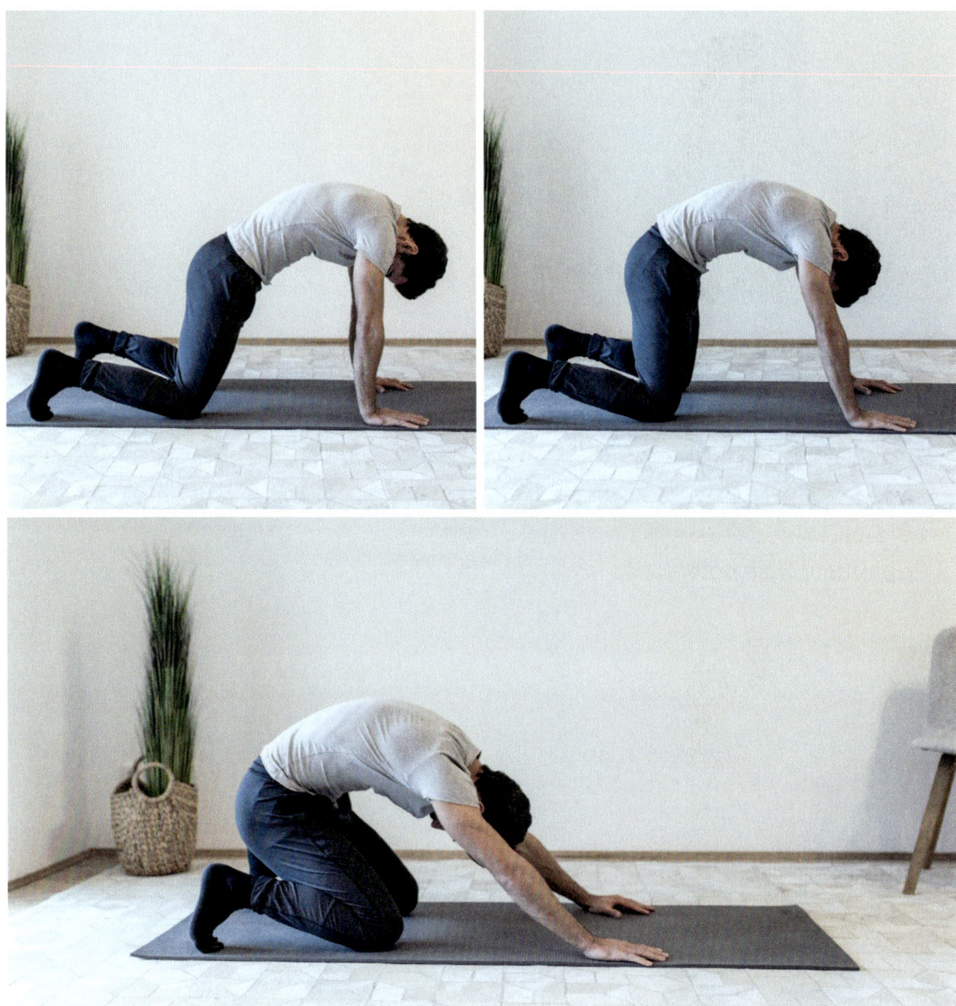

Fig. 3.21: Back breathing (back and forth two times)

Start on all fours. Position the hands under the shoulders. Push your hands against the floor so that you round your upper back and move the shoulder blades apart. Breathe two or three full breaths into this stretched area before you move your hips back a bit. Feel how the stretch in your back moves down to the middle of your spine as you work to keep your spine rounded as much as possible. Stay here and breathe another two or three full breaths into the stretched area. Next move the hips all the way back. In this position, feel the stretch in the lower back, breathing into this area again. Then repeat the same steps in the reverse order. Go slowly, and if you feel too much discomfort, stay in the positions that feel more comfortable.

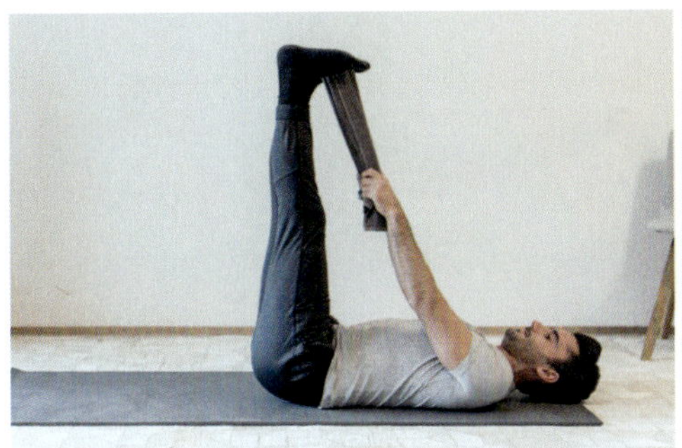
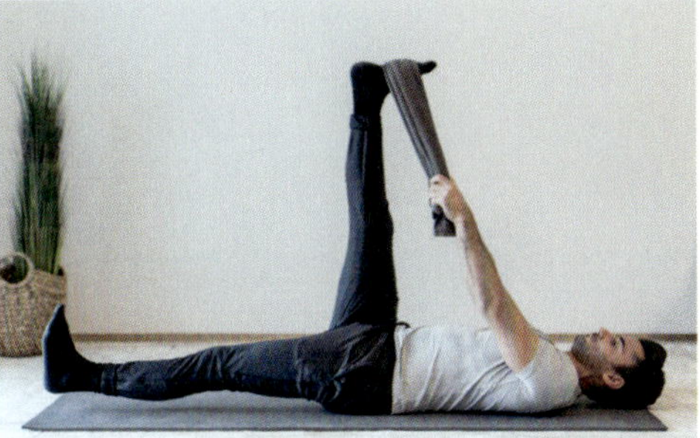

Fig. 3.22: Leg lower with towel (10 reps)

Lie on your back and lift your legs toward the ceiling. Hold one leg up with the help of a towel. Next lower the opposite leg toward the floor and then lift it again. The farther down you lower the leg, the greater the stretch is in the back of the raised leg. With each repetition, try to lower the leg a bit farther while holding the raised leg in its position. Train both sides and repeat on the side that feels tighter.

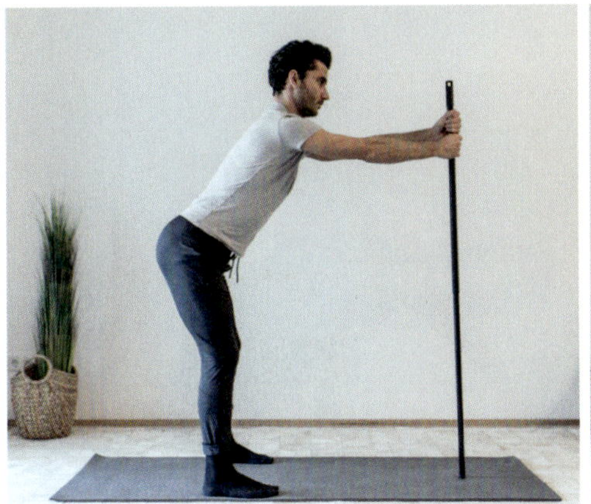
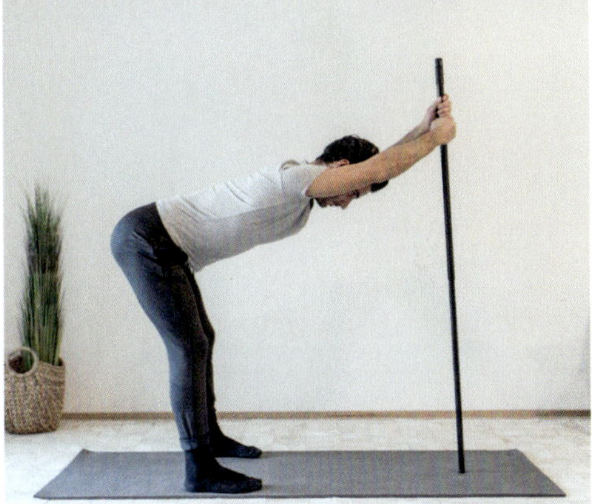

Fig. 3.23: Hip hinge stretch with stick (hold for 10 breaths)

Stand with feet hip-width apart and facing forward. Hinge forward, keeping the back completely straight and stretching the arms out while pressing the stick down into the floor. Then let your upper body sink down to the lowest point in which you can still maintain a straight spine. This is done in order to create a greater stretch in your hamstrings and shoulders.

With every inhalation, work to move the stick forward and the hips backward, and with the exhalation, work to maintain the length in your whole body.

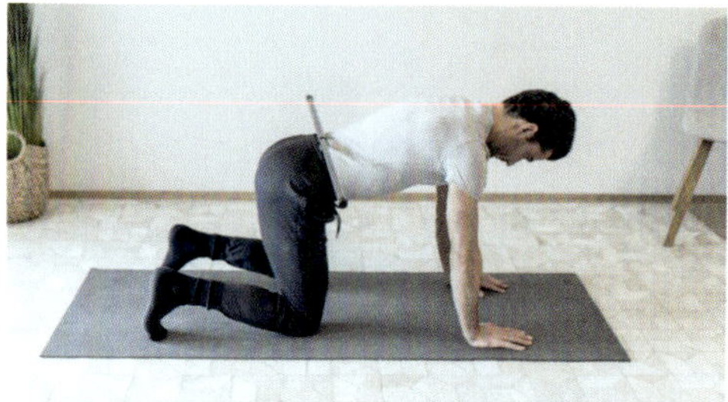

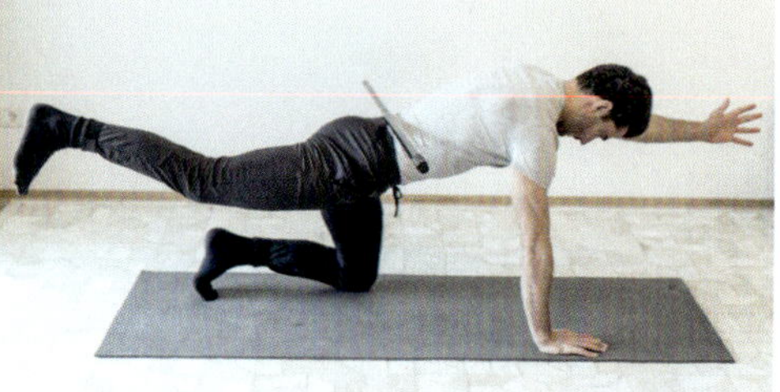

Fig. 3.24: Bird dog with stick (5 x 5-second hold)

On all fours, place the stick across your back. Position your hands under your shoulders and your knees under your hips, keeping your spine in a neutral position.

Now, as you exhale, stretch one arm forward at shoulder level while stretching the opposite leg behind with the foot flexed toward your knee. Stay in this position, breathing deeply into your abdomen and lower rib cage and working to keep your torso stable enough to prevent the stick from falling down.

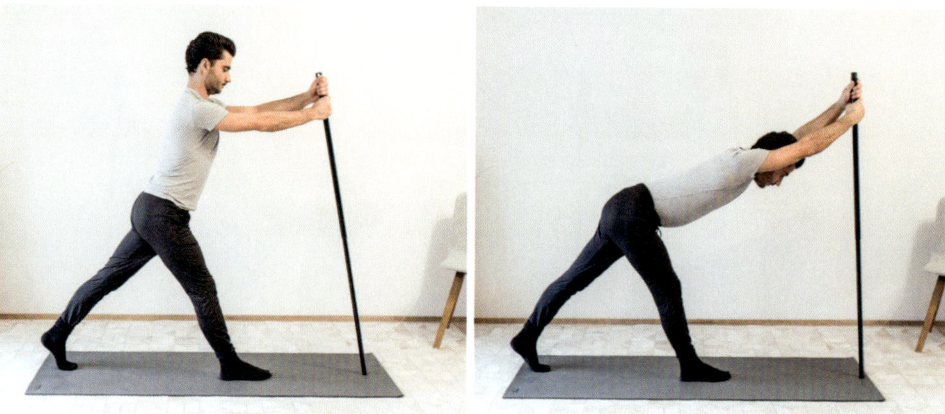

Fig. 3.25: Single-leg hip hinge with stick (hold for 10 breaths)

Come to a short lunge position in which your front leg is mostly straight with only a minimal bend in the knee and your rear leg is completely stretched with the heel lifted. Hinge forward from the hips and lower your upper body as far as possible while keeping your back straight. If your back begins to round, you've gone too far. You want to feel a stretch in the hamstring, glute, and calf muscles of the front leg. Next, when you stretch your arms, press the stick into the floor with moderate pressure. Work to expand your rib cage three-dimensionally while inhaling and elongating your body from feet to hands.

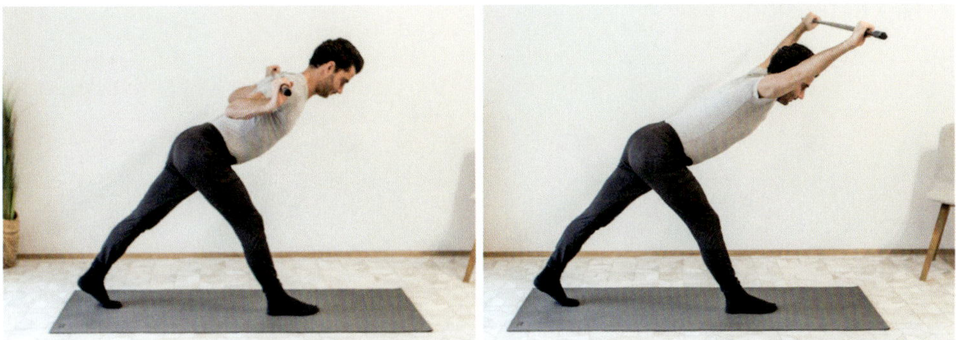

Fig. 3.26: Single-leg hip hinge with stick raised (hold for 10 breaths)

Come to a short lunge position with the front leg mostly straight with only minimal bend in the knee, and your rear leg is completely stretched with the heel lifted. Hold the stick across your back at shoulder level and hinge forward from the hips. Lower your upper body as far as you can while still keeping your back straight. Finally, stretch your arms out forward with your palms facing down and work to pull the stick apart. Stay in this position. Breathe three-dimensionally and elongate your body from feet to hands.

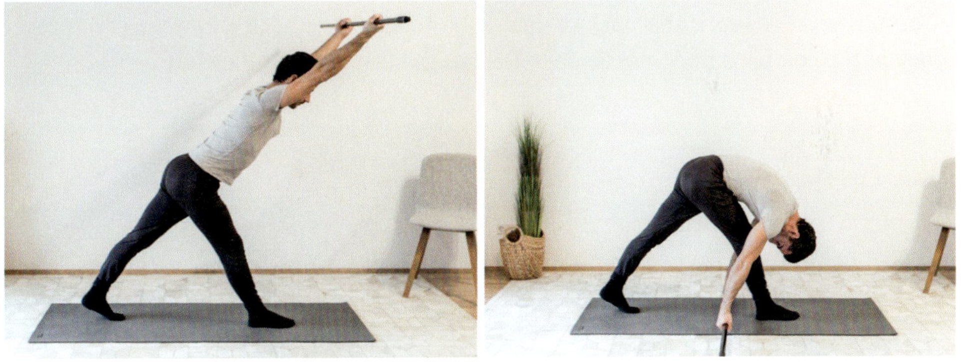

Fig. 3.27: Single-leg forward fold with stick (hold for 10 breaths)

Come to a short lunge position, keeping your front leg straight with only minimal bend in the knee, and your rear leg completely stretched with the heel lifted. With palms facing up, straighten your arms, pushing the stick overhead. Hinge forward from the hips, bending as far as possible and rounding your spine. If you can bend far enough, step over the stick with your front leg and push it toward your rear leg. Stay in this position or bounce back and forth slightly, activating the facia in your whole superficial back line.

2. Hip Extension:

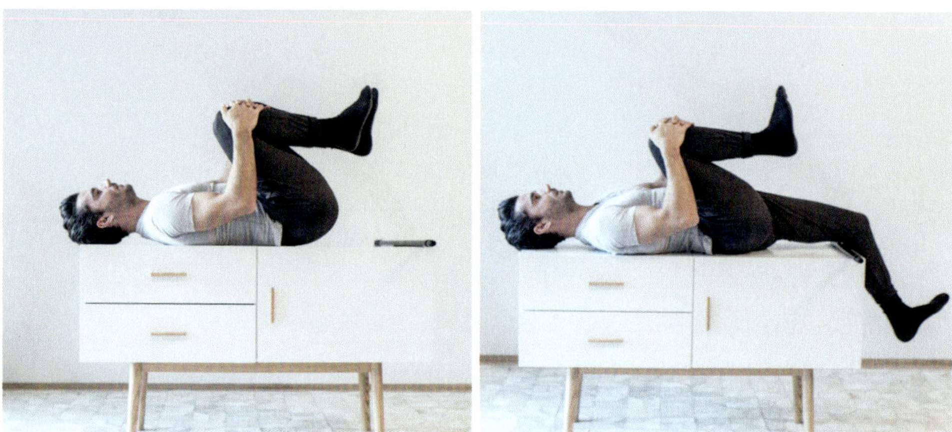

Fig. 3.28: Testing hip extension mobility

Lie on the edge of a table so that the backs of your knees are in line with the edge of the table and position the stick right on that edge under your knees. Pull both knees toward you and hold them up with your hands. Then lower one leg slowly until the back of the knee touches the stick while the knee is bent.

You passed this test if the back of your knee touches the stick without performing any of the compensatory movements. Repeat the test on the other side.

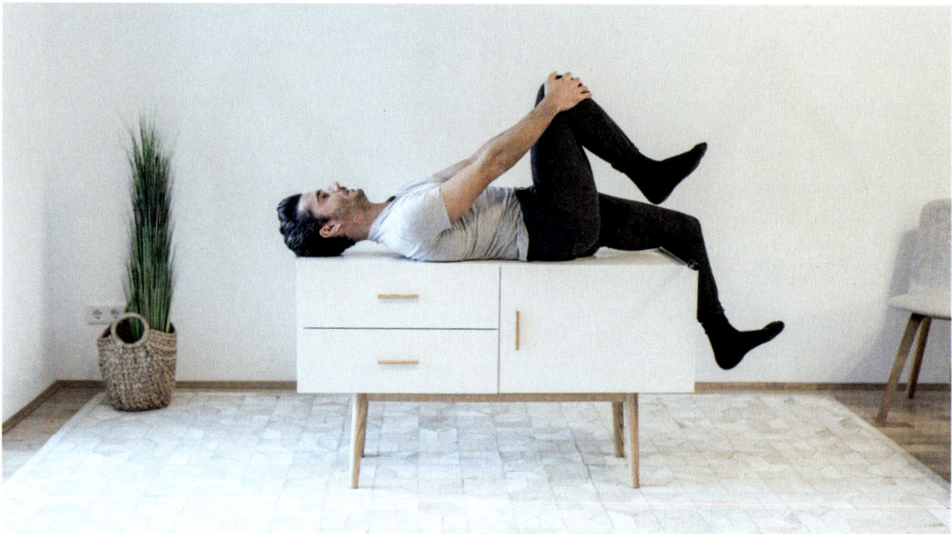

Fig. 3.29: Compensation 1: Moving the leg that is pulled into the chest forward

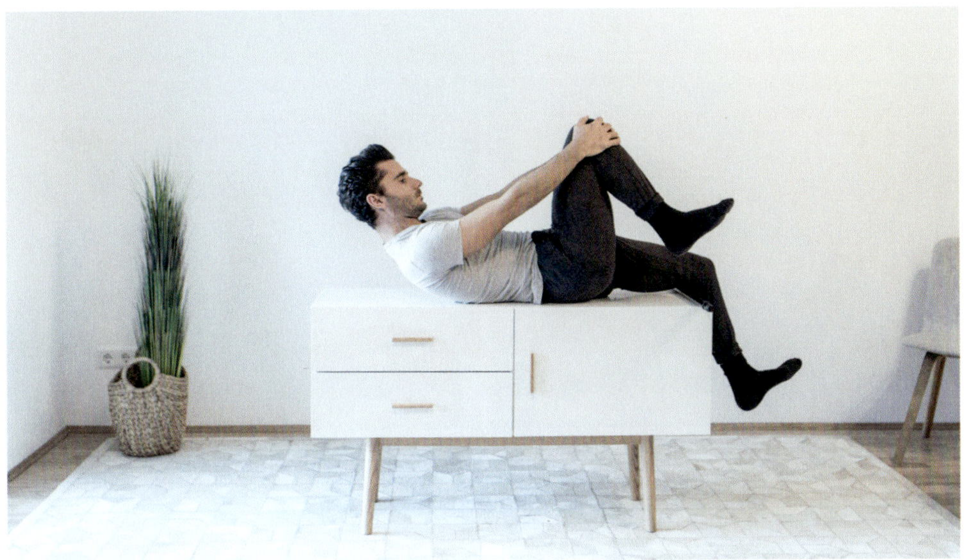

Fig. 3.30: Compensation 2: Lifting the head and shoulders

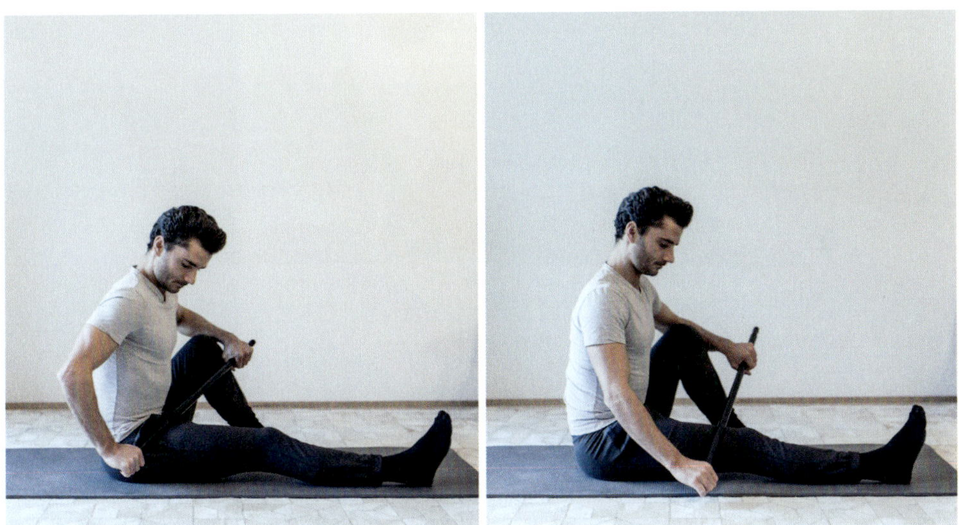

Fig. 3.31: Treating the fascia of the thighs (1 minute per side)

Sit upright on the floor with one leg pulled toward the butt and the other one stretched out. Place the stick across the thigh of the straight leg and move it back and forth rapidly, from the hip down to right above the kneecap. Apply more stroking and pressure to areas that feel more uncomfortable, but do so gently so that no pain occurs. If this position is too uncomfortable for your back you can also sit on a chair.

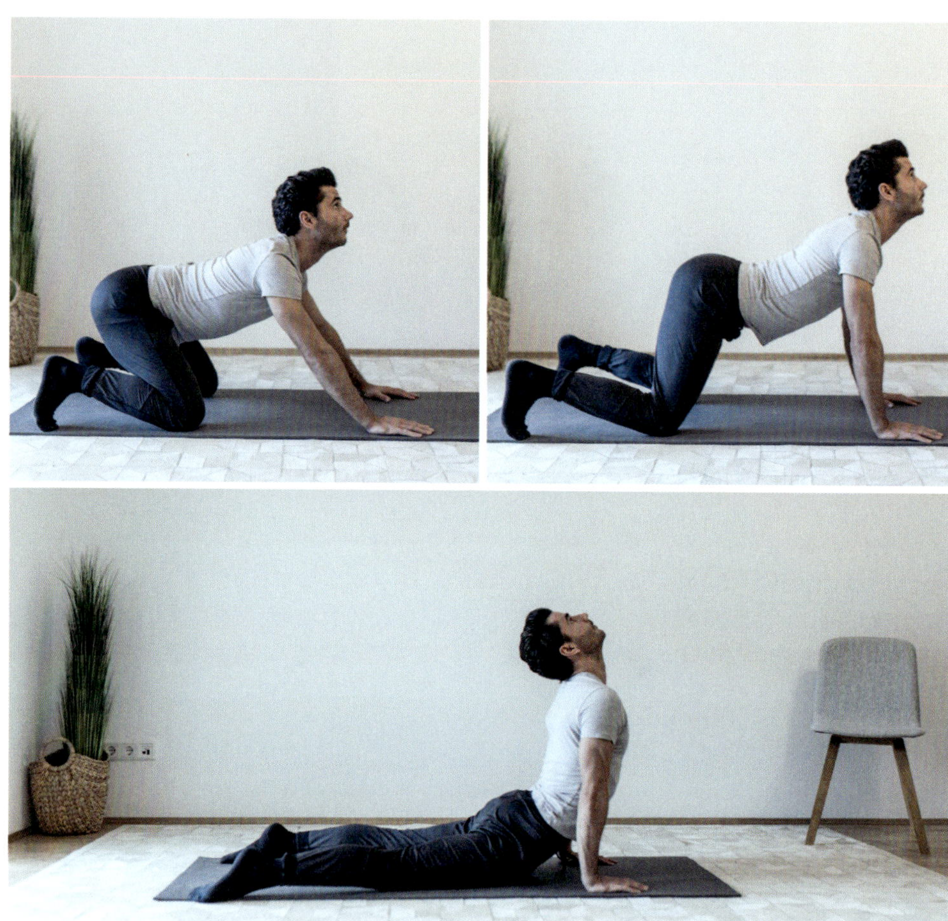

Fig. 3.32: Front breathing (back and forth two times)

Start on all fours. Begin pressing the hips back as far as possible toward the heels, while working to arch your back as much as possible and bringing your shoulder blades together. Breathe two to three times into your chest and belly, feeling them open with every inhalation. Next, move your hips forward until your shoulders are back in line with your hands. Hold this position and breathe two to three times into the whole front side of your body. Feel how the stretch moves down toward the stomach. Finally, move the hips all the way forward and down while you extend the arms and lift the gaze high. In this position, feel the stretch mainly in your abdominal muscles. Breathe into this area again. Move slowly back to the starting position. If you feel too much pressure in your lower back, stay in the positions that feel more comfortable.

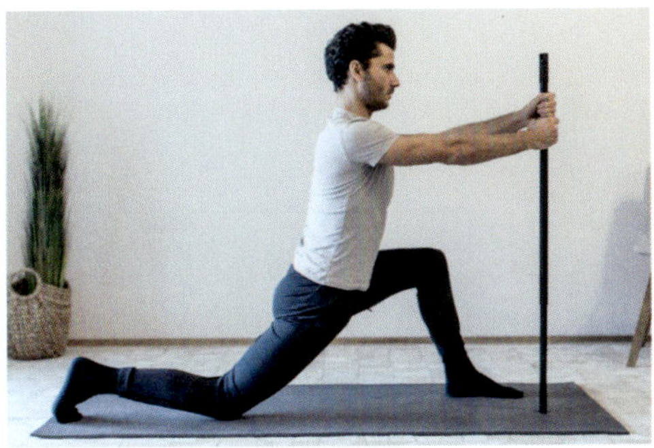
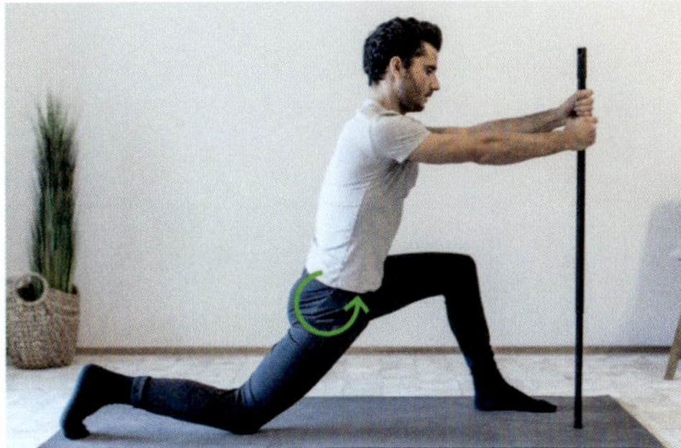

Fig. 3.33: Hip flexor stretch with stick (hold for 10 breaths)

Stand in a kneeling lunge position, with a right angle in the front leg and the rear toes curled under. Hold the stick vertically in front of you and press it into the ground. With your whole spine straight, tilt your pelvis up and back and let it sink down. Tense your gluteal muscles and feel the stretch in the front of your extended back leg. Stay in this position and breathe deeply into your abdomen and lower rib cage so that they expand in all directions. After completing the stretch on both sides, train the side that feels stiffer again.

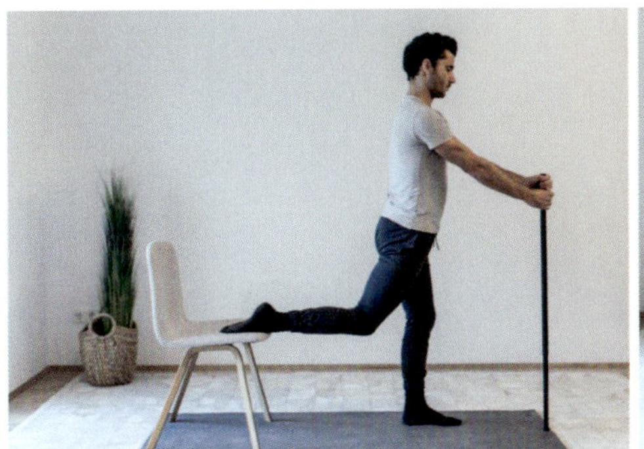
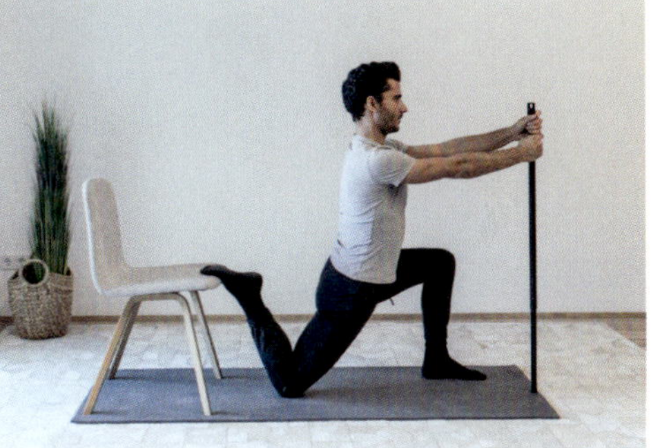

Fig. 3.34: Hip flexor stretch with elevated rear foot (hold for 10 breaths)

Position the top of your foot on a chair that's behind you, and keep the other foot on the floor, with your ankle directly underneath your knee. Hold the stick vertically and press it down into the floor. Next, slowly bend your front leg until your back knee is on the floor, while keeping your spine completely straight. Afterward, tilt your pelvis up and back, so that your gluteal muscles are tensed and you feel a stretch in the front thigh of the back leg. Stay in this position and breathe deeply into your abdomen and lower rib cage so that they expand in all directions. After completing the stretch on both sides, train the side that feels stiffer again.

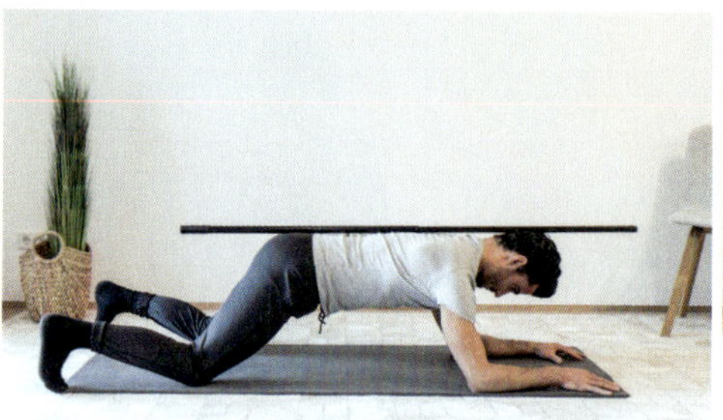
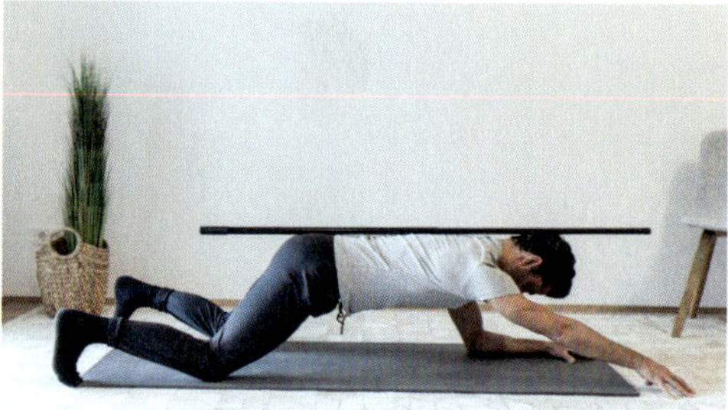

Fig. 3.35: Plank with arm slide (10 reps each side)

Start on your stomach and position the stick along your spine so that it has contact with your butt, upper back, and head. Then bring your elbows underneath your shoulders and push up so that only your elbows, hands, feet, and knees touch the floor. Keep your palms facing down. Your entire spine should be in a neutral position, with your elbows slightly in front of your shoulders and your knees well behind your pelvis. Then, as you exhale, slide one arm forward, lifting the elbow while trying to keep your pelvis and core stable enough to prevent the stick from falling.

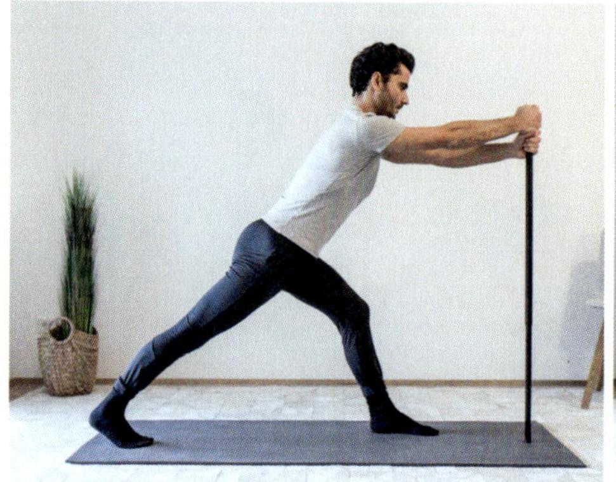
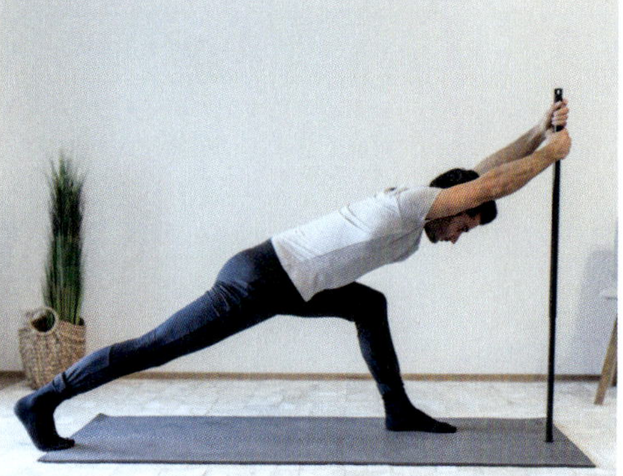

Fig. 3.36: Lunge hinge with stick (hold for 10 breaths)

Get into a long lunge position. Stretch the arms out and press the stick into the floor, using moderate pressure. Tilt your pelvis up and back, letting it sink down so that you feel a stretch in the front of your extended back leg. Next, bring your upper body down to the point where you can still maintain a straight back. Try to push your back heel as far back as possible while pushing the stick forward and down, straightening the arms. Stay in this position and expand your rib cage three-dimensionally while inhaling, elongating your body from feet to hands.

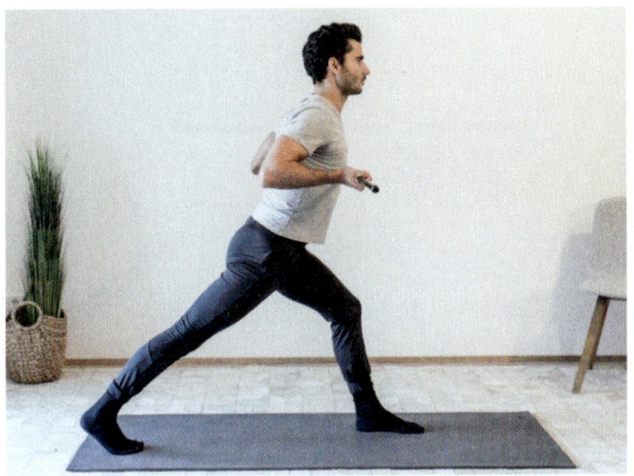

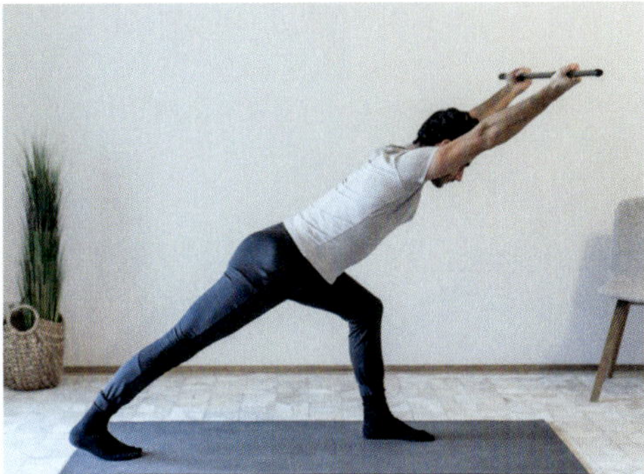

Fig. 3.37: Lunge hinge with stick raised (hold for 10 breaths)

Get into a long lunge position, and hold the stick in front of you at chest level. Tilt your pelvis up and back, letting it sink down so that you feel a stretch in the front of your extended back leg. Then bring your upper body down to the point where you can still maintain a straight back and stretch your arms out forward with your palms facing up. Try to pull the stick apart gently while still keeping your arms up as high as possible. Stay in this position, breathing three-dimensionally and elongating your body from feet to hands.

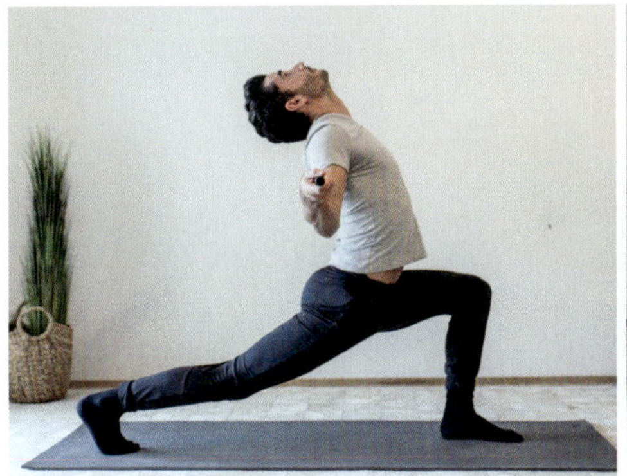

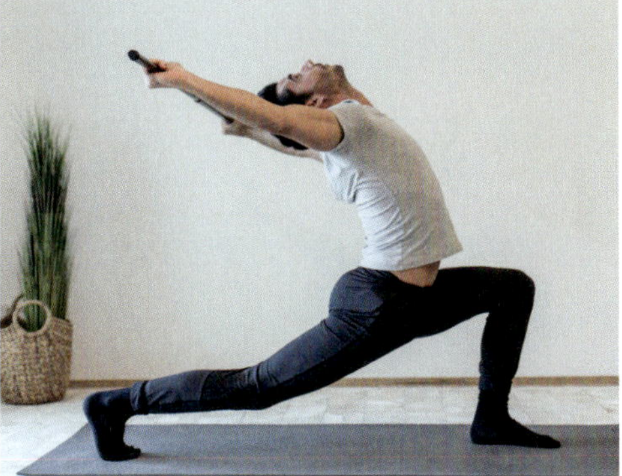

Fig. 3.38: Lunge hinge with back bend (hold for 10 breaths)

Get into a long lunge position, holding the stick up over your head and creating tension by pulling it apart gently. Tilt your pelvis up and back, letting it sink down so that you feel a stretch in the front of your extended back leg. Squeezing the glutes together, arch back as far as you can. Stay in this position and try to breath as deeply as possible, feeling an even greater stretch when breathing in and elongating the front of your body.

3. Rib Cage Control

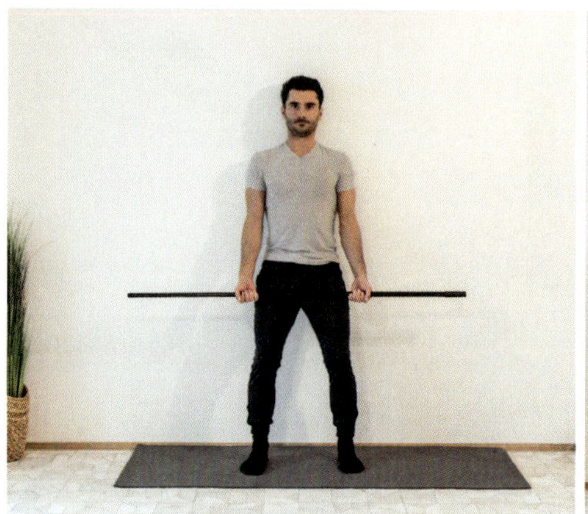
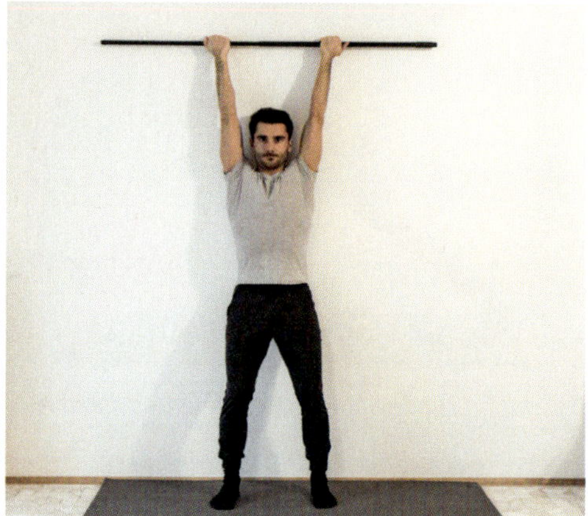

Fig. 3.39: Testing rib cage motor control

Stand with your back against a wall. Hold the stick shoulder-width apart and with your palms facing forward in front of you. Bend your knees slightly and tilt your pelvis posteriorly so that your whole back is touching the wall. Then move the stick above your head until your fingers touch the wall while your arms stay completely stretched. You have passed this test when your fingers touch the wall with arms completely stretched, and you haven't performed any compensatory movements.

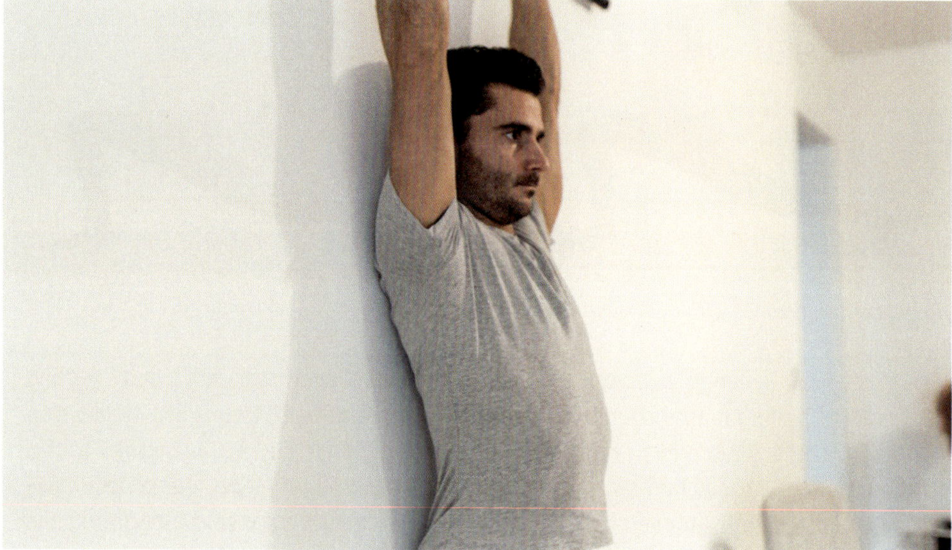

Fig. 3.40: Compensation 1: Back loses contact with the wall

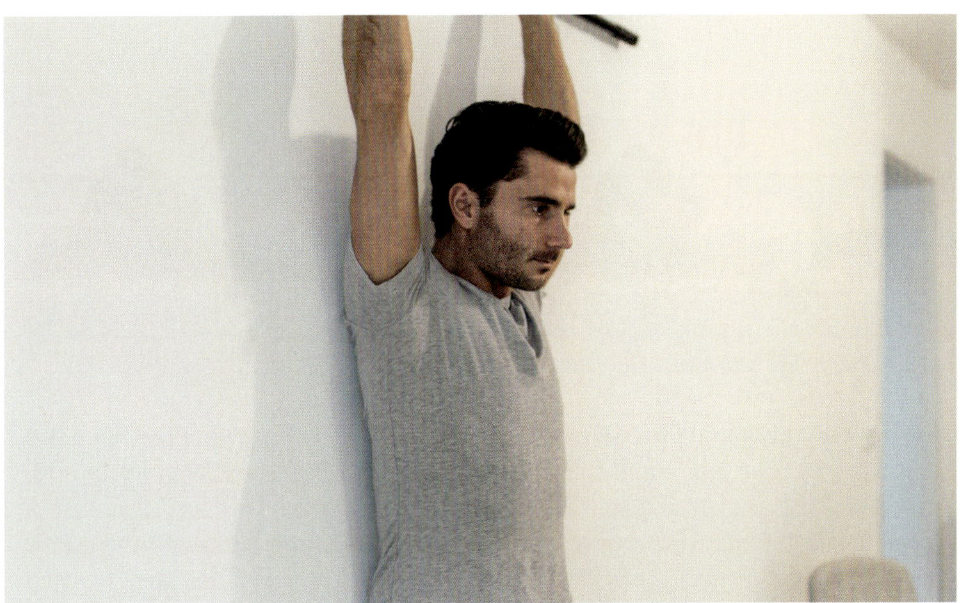

Fig. 3.41: Compensation 2: Head moves forward

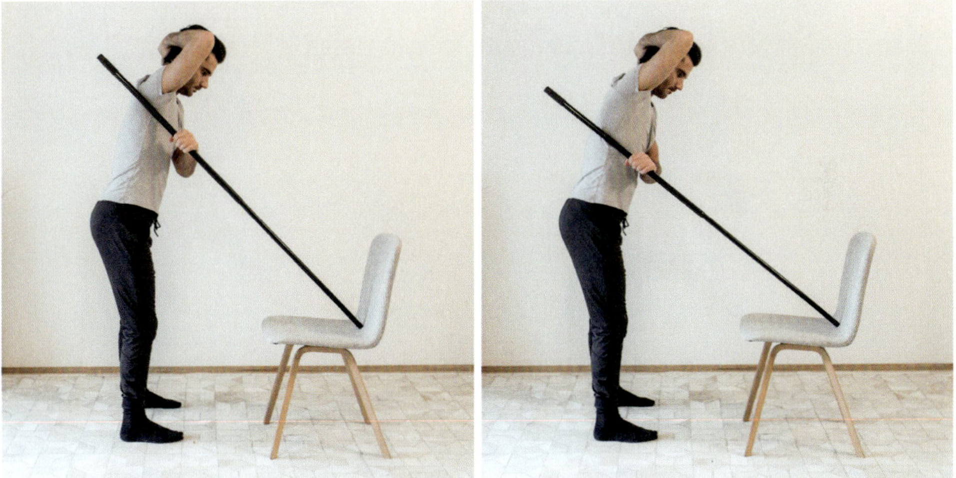

Fig. 3.42: Treating the fascia of the outer rib cage

Stand in front of a chair and position the stick on the lower end of the chair at an angle. Place one hand on the back of your head and use the hand on the opposite side of the stick to apply pressure the muscles that run from right below your arm pit to the bottom of your rib cage by using rapid up and down movements. Apply additional pressure to areas that feel uncomfortable, but not so much that there is pain.

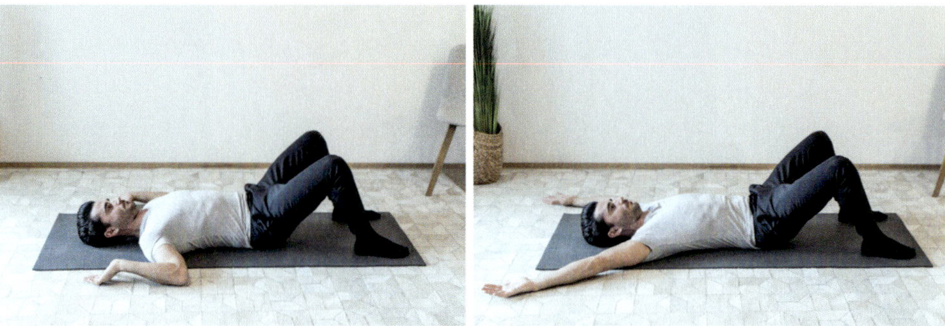

Fig. 3.43: Arm slide with focus on exhalation (2 x 5 breaths)

Lie on your back with your knees bent and your legs engaged. Tilt your pelvis backward so that your entire spine connects with the floor. Next, bring your arms into a W position, keeping your hands and elbows against the floor. Then, take a deep breath through your nose and into your belly and lower rib cage so that they expand in all directions. Then blow the air out completely as if you were blowing through a straw while sliding your arms diagonally overhead along the floor. Lower your rib cage so that your back is completely touching the floor. When you have completely exhaled, hold your breath for three seconds. The subsequent inhalation is again through your nose while your mouth remains closed.

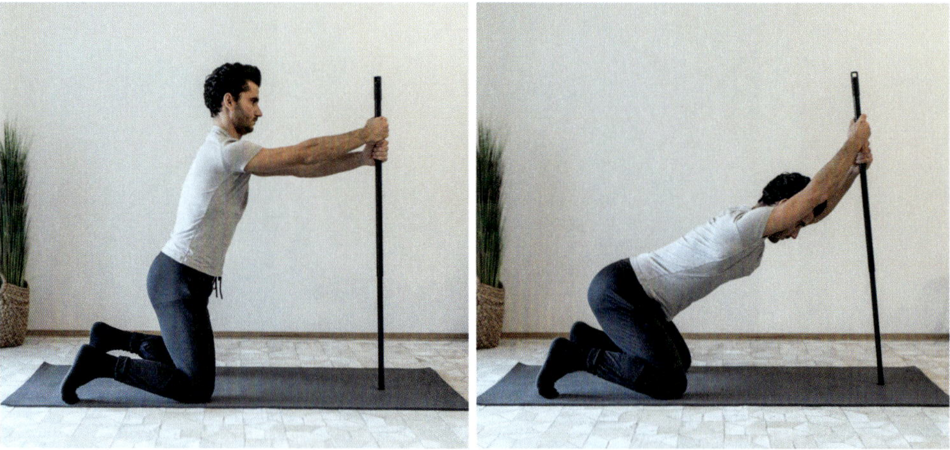

Fig. 3.44: Kneeling shoulder stretch with stick (hold for 10 breaths)

Get into a kneeling position and place the stick on the floor in front of you with your arms outstretched. Then lower your upper body while trying to push the stick forward and pulling the butt back to elongate your entire upper body.

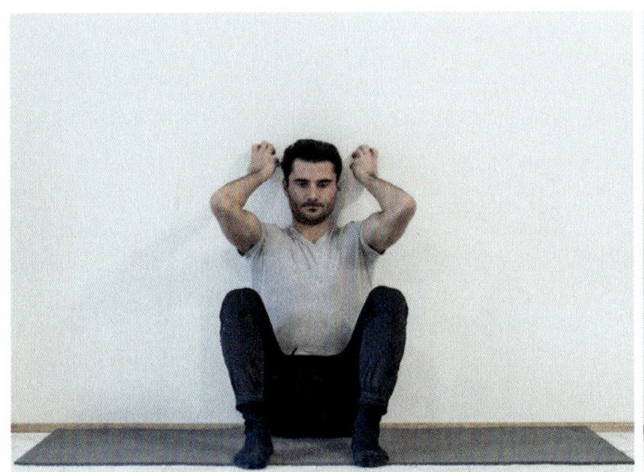
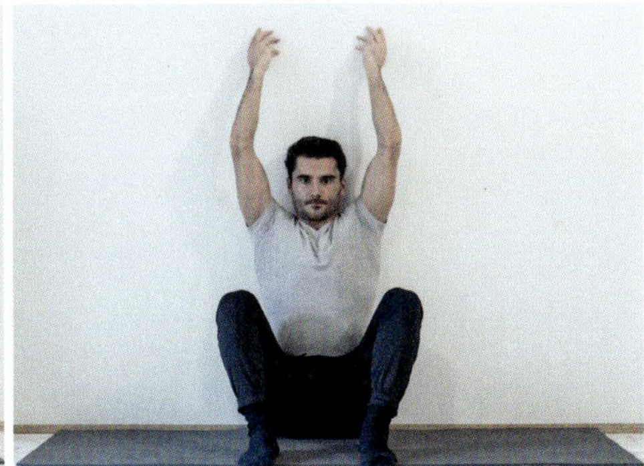

Fig. 3.45: Finger slide on wall (2 x 5 reps)

Sit with your back against a wall and pull your feet back toward your butt. Place your arms next to your head, keeping your elbows forward and your fingertips pressed against the wall. Then inhale deeply into your stomach and lower rib cage. As you exhale, bring your hands up as far as you can while you still keep your back and fingers pressed against the wall. Exhale completely in the final position until you feel slight tension in your abdominal muscles.

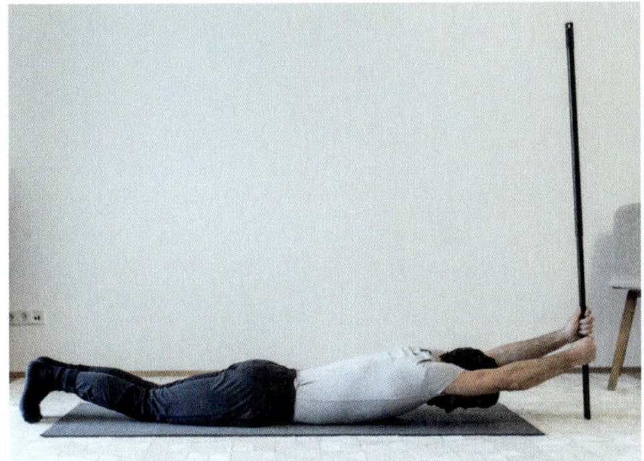
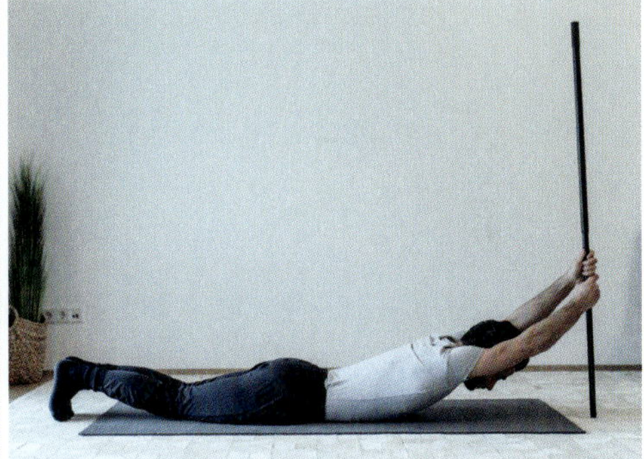

Fig. 3.46: Prone thoracic extension with stick (hold for 10 breaths)

Lie on your stomach. Stretch out your arms and press the stick down gently into the floor. Your knees should be together and touching the floor while your feet are flexed. Then try to grab the stick at the highest point possible. The stick should stay perpendicular to the floor the whole time.

Breathe in to expand your rib cage three-dimensionally while pushing the stick forward. When you breathe out, try to keep the length in your spine to engage your core muscles.

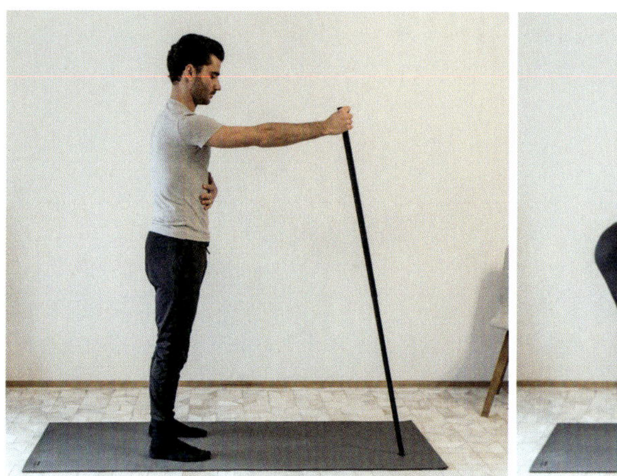

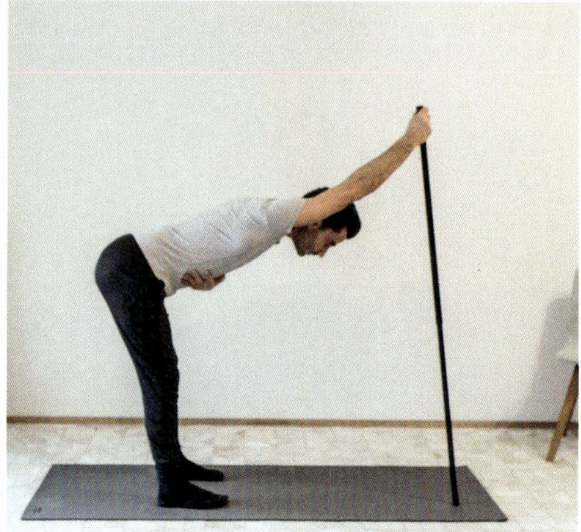

Fig. 3.47: Single-arm hip hinge with stick (hold for 10 breaths)

Stand with feet hip-width apart and press the stick into the floor, keeping the arms straight. Bend your legs slightly and hinge forward to the point where you can feel a stretch in your hamstrings but still maintain a straight spine.

Hold the stick in one hand and place the other hand on the rib cage as a check that the ribs are not flaring out (moving forward), which would mean you're overextending your back.

With every inhalation, try to move the stick forward and the hips backward. With every exhalation, try to maintain that length along your whole body.

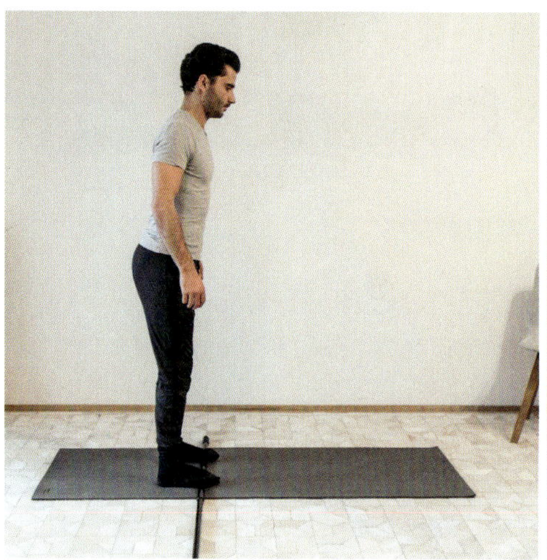

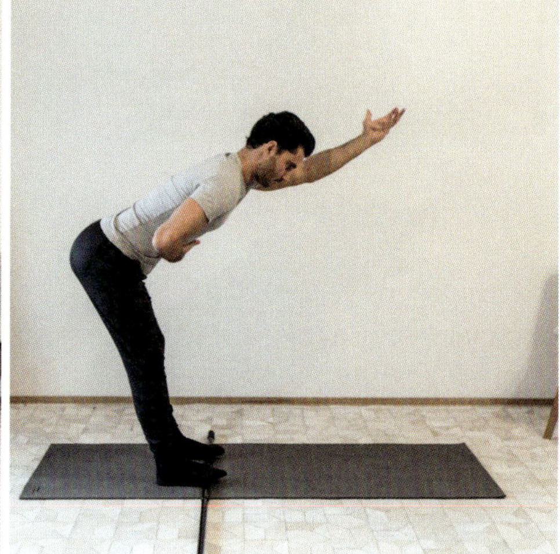

Fig. 3.48: Hip hinge with single-arm raise (hold for 10 breaths)

Stand with feet hip-width apart the balls of your feet on the stick. Bend the legs slightly and hinge forward as far as you can while so that you feel a stretch in the hamstrings but can still maintain a straight spine.

Then, with palm facing the ceiling, move one arm forward and up as high as possible. The other hand is on the rib cage, making sure the ribs do not flair out (move forward), overextending the back.

With every inhalation, try to move the stick forward and the hips backward, and with the exhalation, try to maintain that length in your whole body.

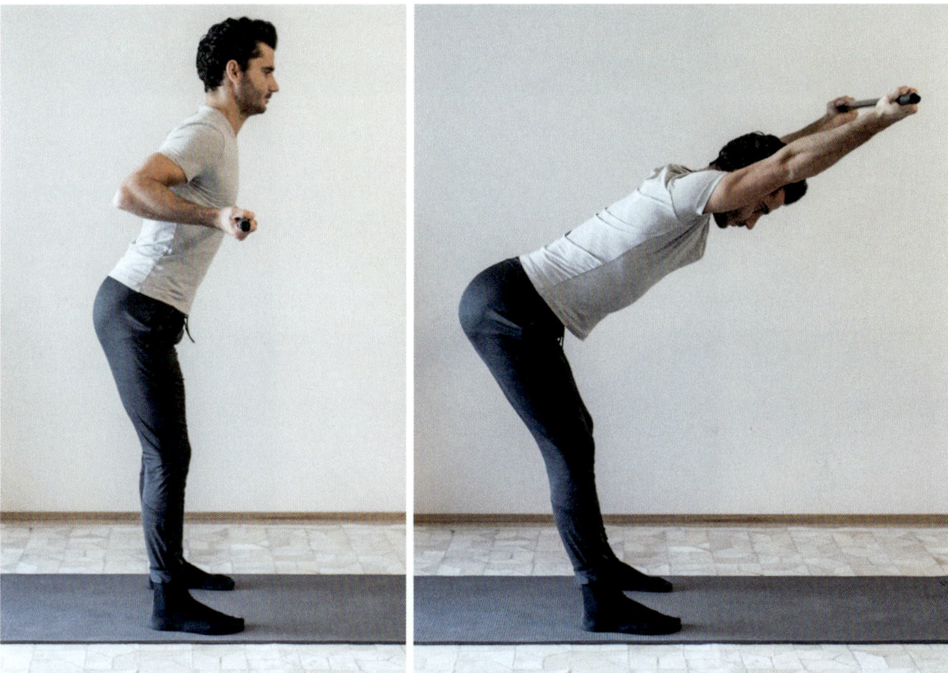

Fig. 3.49: Hip hinge with stick raised (hold for 10 breaths)

Stand in a hip-width position. Hold the stick slightly wider than shoulder-width apart with palms facing up in front of you. Bend the legs slightly and hinge forward to the point where you can feel a stretch in your hamstrings while still maintaining a straight spine. At the same time, move the arms forward and up as high as possible, pulling the stick apart slightly.

Stay in this position and breathe deeply into your core and lower rib cage so that they expand in all directions.

4. External Hip Rotation

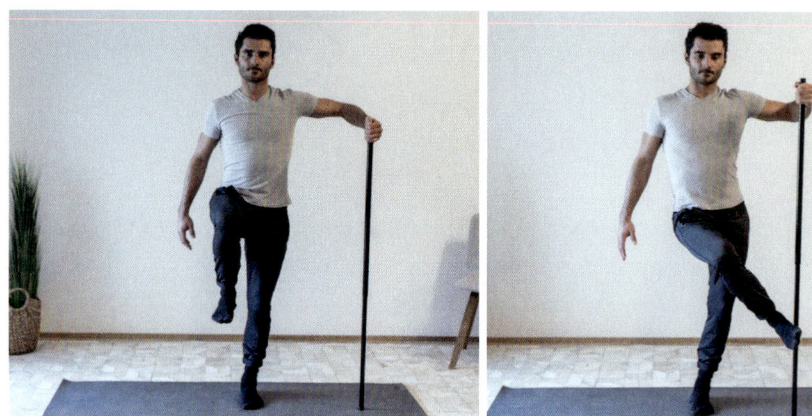

Fig. 3.50: Testing hip external rotation mobility

Stand upright, holding the stick next to you with a 90-degree bend in the arm. Press the stick gently into the floor while lifting the leg on the opposite side to a 90-degree angle so that the knee is in line with the hip. Move the foot toward the stick until the heel touches it. You have passed this test when your heel touches the stick without performing any of the compensatory movements. Repeat the test on the other side as well.

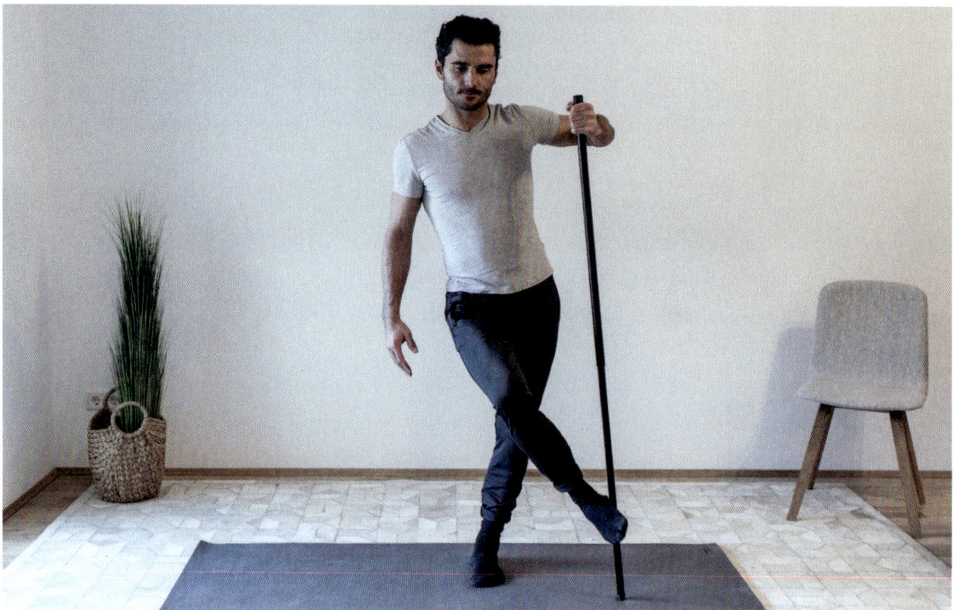

Fig. 3.51: Compensation 1: Moving the stick toward you

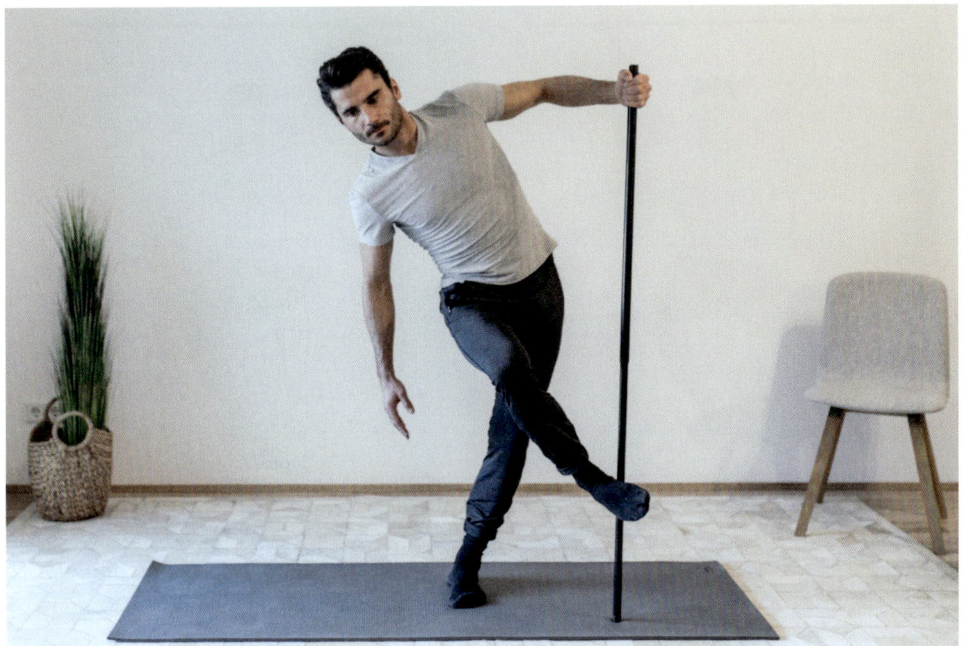

Fig. 3.52: Compensation 2: Tilting the upper body

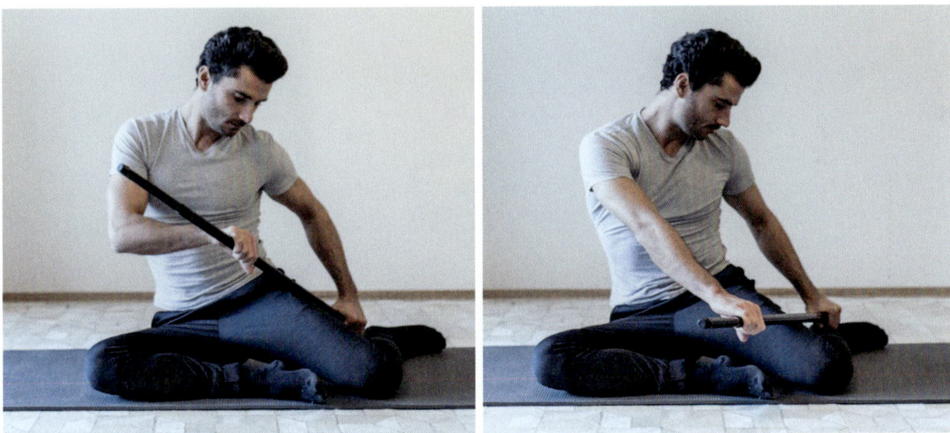

Fig. 3.53: Treating the fascia of the outer thighs (1 minute per side)

Sit up tall with one leg bent in front of you and the other on your side so that the foot is behind you. Place the stick across the outside of the thigh and move it rapidly back and forth from the hip down to right above the knee. Apply more pressure in areas that feel more uncomfortable, but not so much that you feel pain. If this position is too uncomfortable for you, do the movements while standing.

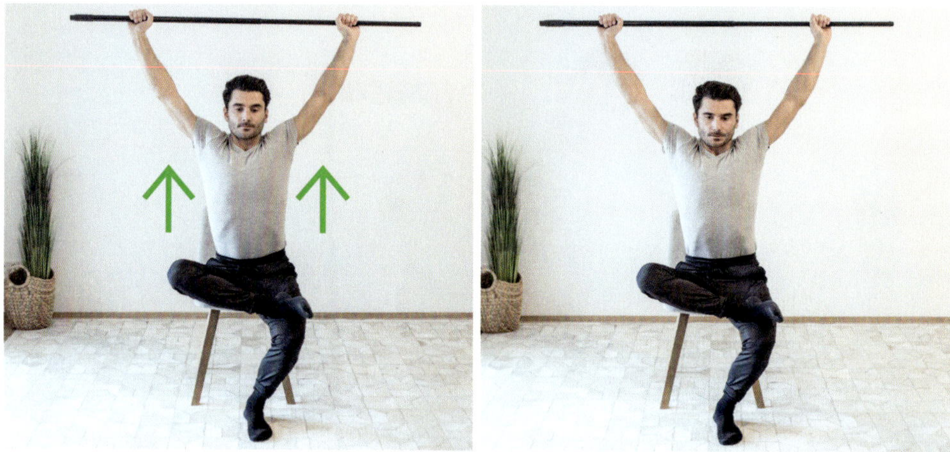

Fig. 3.54: Breathing with rib cage lift on chair (2 x 5 breaths)

Sit on a chair. Position one foot on the opposite thigh and hold the stick over your head. Pull the stick apart slightly and bring your head back so it's aligned with the spine. Then breathe in to lift your entire rib cage, front and back, up as much as possible while you push the knee of your upper leg down gently. When you breathe out, try to maintain the length in your spine, feeling how the core is engaged.

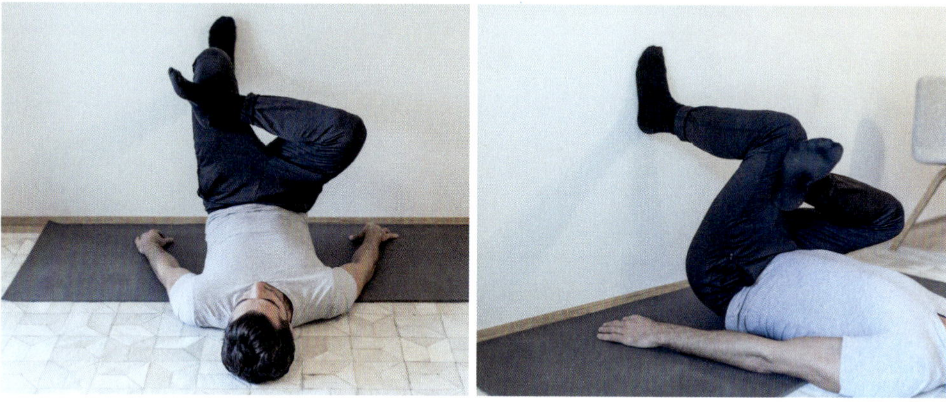

Fig. 3.55: Outer hip stretch on wall (hold for 10 breaths)

Lie in front of a wall and position your feet on it so that you have a 90-degree angle in your hips as well as your knees. Then lift your hips up slightly and place one foot on top of the opposite leg's thigh. Push your knee toward the wall, lowering your butt back down slowly, feeling an increased stretching sensation in the glutes of your upper leg.

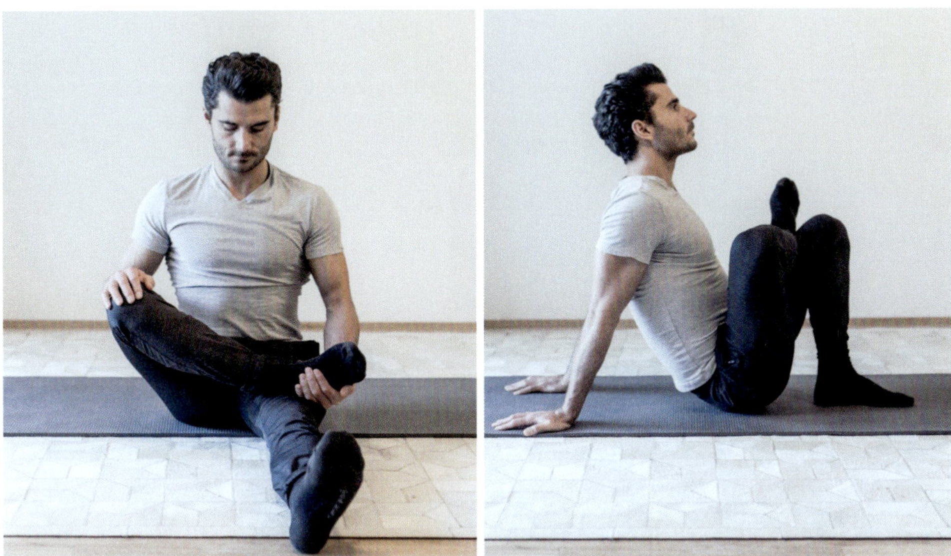

Fig. 3.56: Sitting outer hip stretch (hold for 10 breaths)

Sit with legs outstretched on the floor and place one foot on top of the opposite leg's thigh. Next, pull the straight leg toward you as far as you can. While you have your hands behind you for support, push the upper knee forward, away from the body, feeling a stretch in the outer hip of that leg.

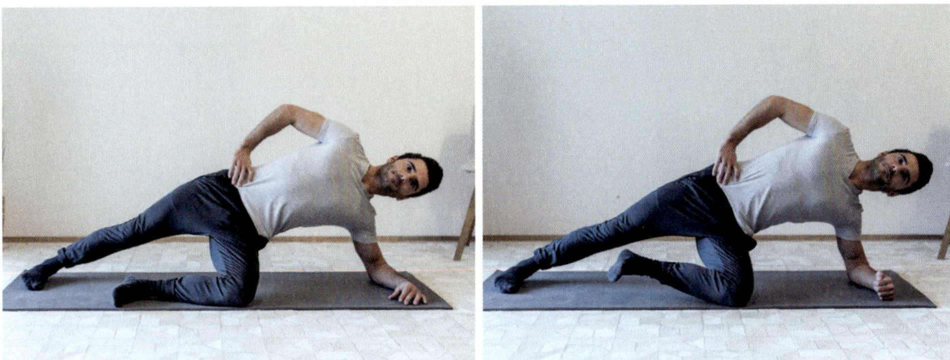

Fig. 3.57: Side plank with external hip rotation (5 reps with 5-second hold)

Come into a side plank position on your elbow. Your lower leg is bent at a 90-degree angle, and your hips are up as high as possible. Keep the knee on the floor and lift the foot up as high as possible. Hold it there for five seconds before lowering it down again.

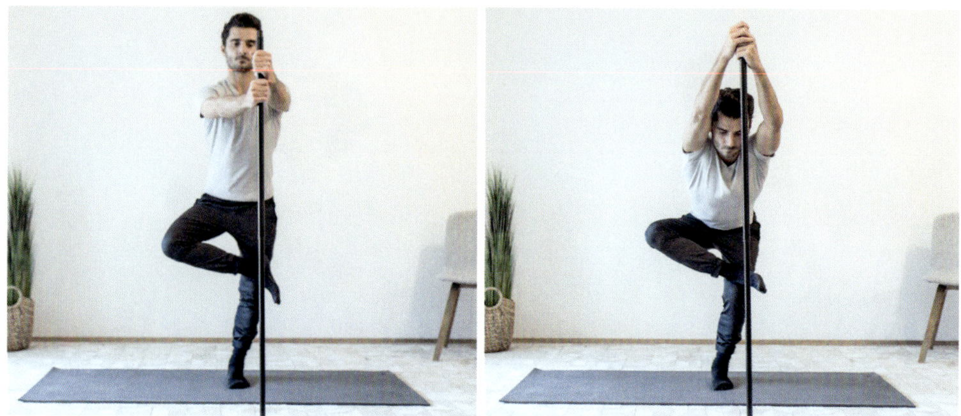

Fig. 3.58: Outer hip hinge with stick (hold for 10 breaths)

Stand upright and place one foot on your opposite leg's thigh. Stretch out your arms and press the stick gently into the floor in front of you. Hinge forward from the hips. Move your hips back as much as possible while pushing the stick forward and down. Lower your upper body to the point where you can still maintain a straight spine and push your upper knee back, activating a stretch in the glutes.

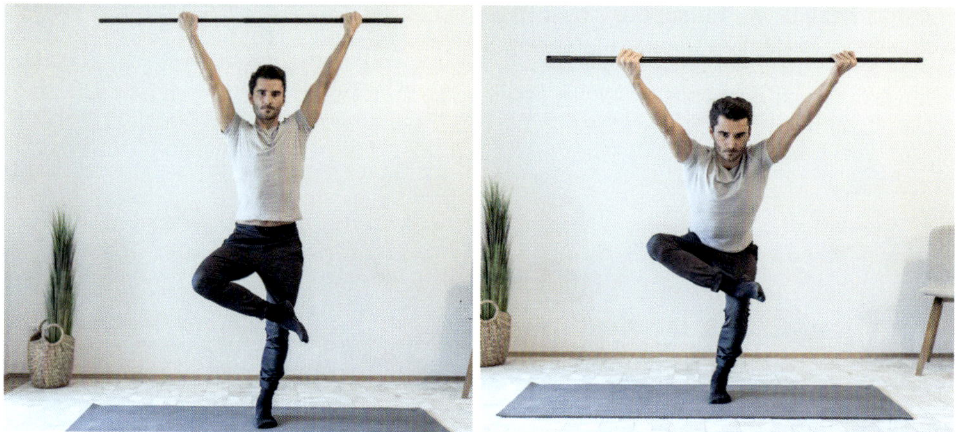

Fig. 3.59: Outer hip hinge with stick raised

Stand upright and place one foot on the opposite leg's thigh. Hold a stick with your hands a bit wider than shoulder-width apart above your head. Keep hands facing up. Then hinge forward and lower your hips slightly by bending your knee. Move your hips back as far as possible while pushing the stick up and forward and your upper knee back, activating a stretch in your glutes.

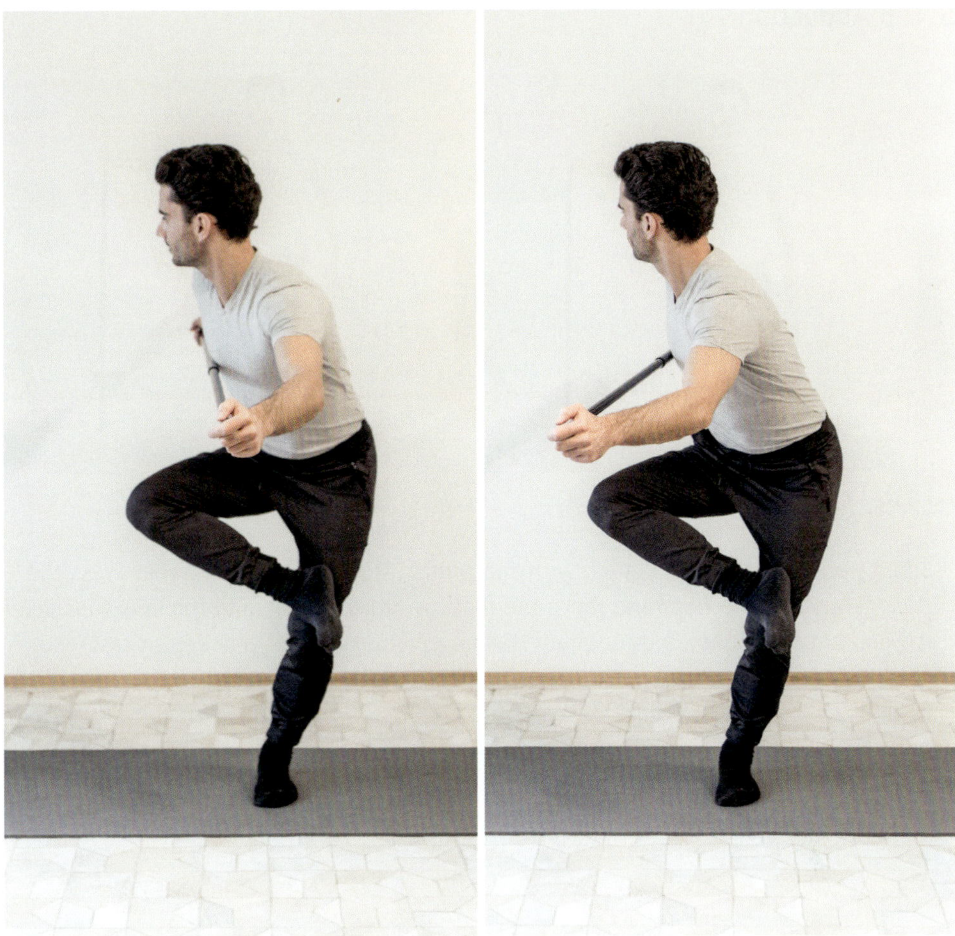

Fig. 3.60: Outer hip hinge with rotation (hold for 10 breaths)

Stand upright and place one foot on your opposite leg's thigh. Hold the stick with your hands a bit wider than shoulder-width apart in front of you.

Then lower your hips slightly and rotate to the side with the lifted leg. With the hand that is in front, push the stick so that it helps you to get even more into the rotation.

5. Hip Abduction

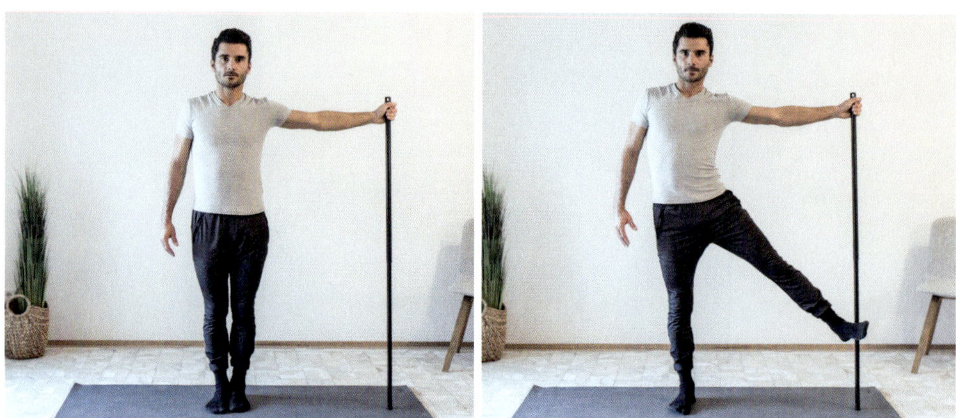

Fig. 3.61: Testing hip abduction mobility

Stand upright, holding the stick with the arm stretched out next to you. Press the stick gently into the floor and move the foot toward the stick until the heel touches it. Maintain a straight leg throughout the movement. You have passed this test when your heel touches the stick without performing any of the compensatory movements. Repeat the test on the other side.

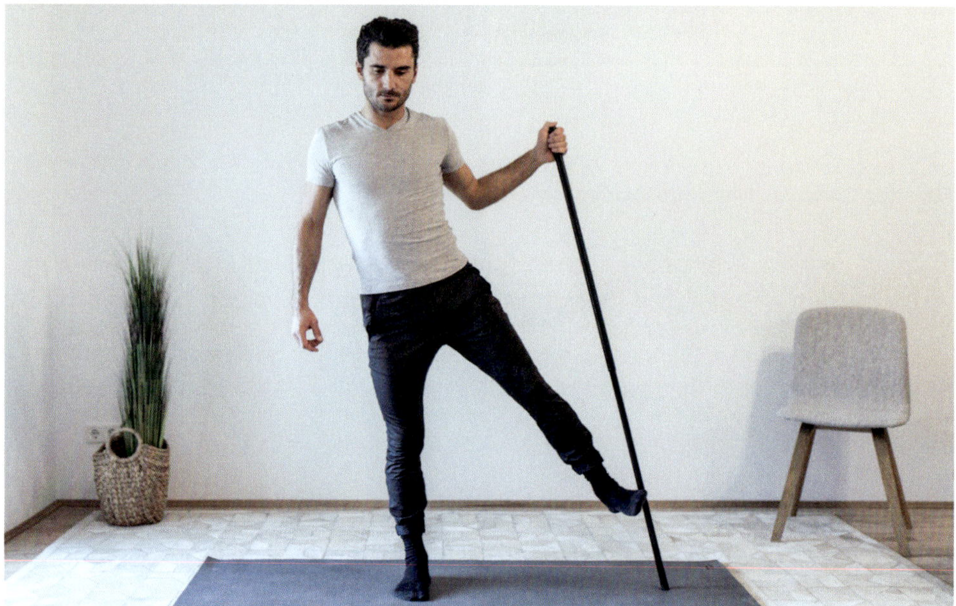

Fig. 3.62: Compensation 1: Moving the stick toward you

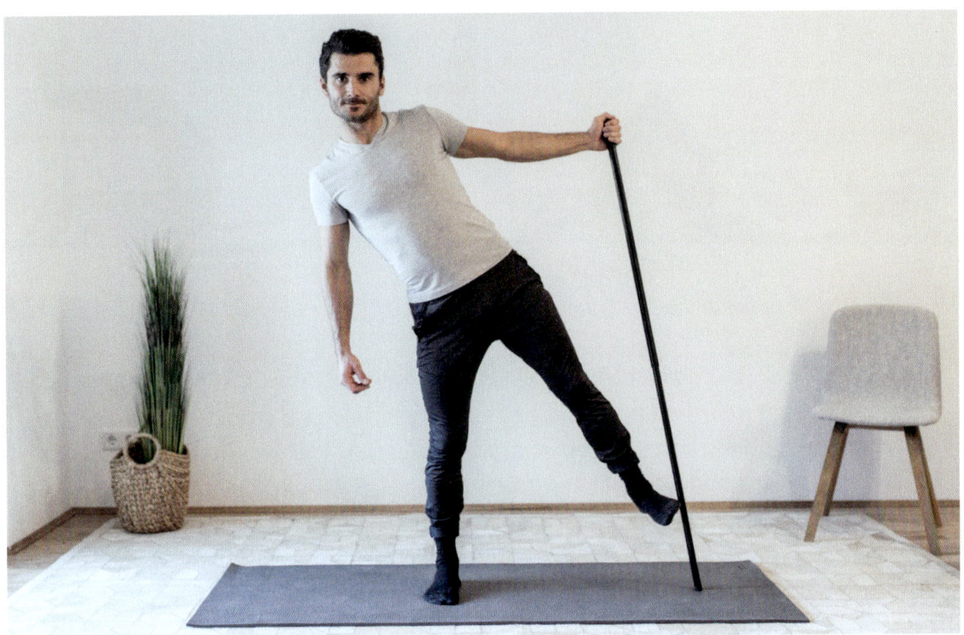

Fig. 3.63: Compensation 2: Tilting the upper body

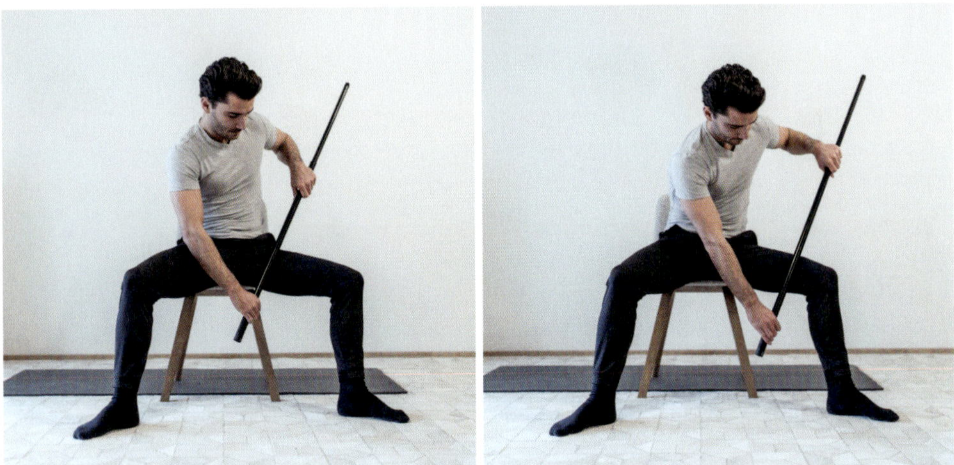

Fig. 3.64: Treating the fascia of the inner thighs (1 minute per side)

Sit on a chair and open your legs wide. Place the stick across your inner thigh and use it to massage the thigh with rapid back-and-forth movements from the hip down to right above the knee. Apply more pressure in areas that feel more uncomfortable, but not so much that you experience pain.

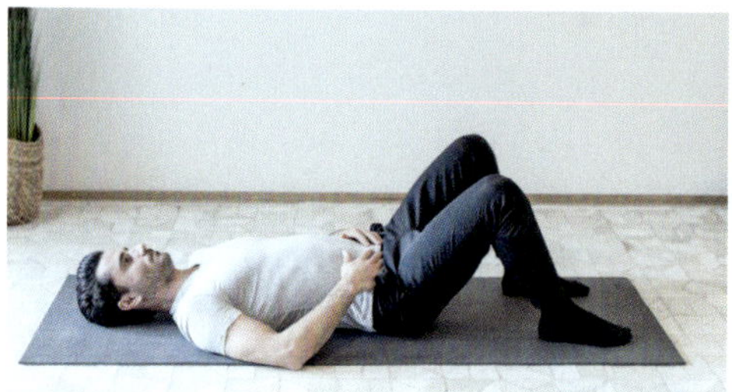
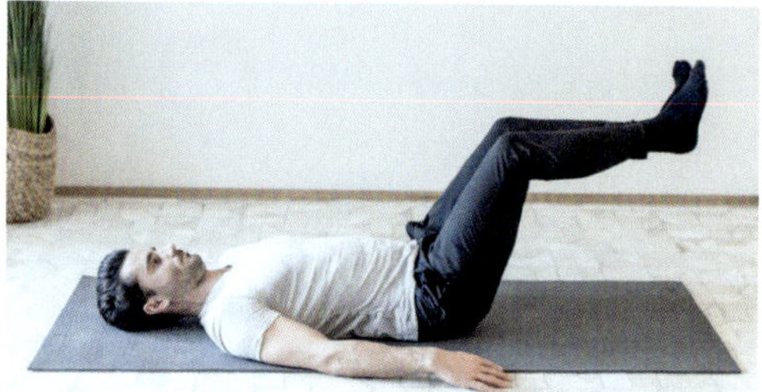

Fig. 3.65: Pelvic floor breathing (2 x 5 breaths)

Lie on your back and place both hands on your lower abdomen. Try to breathe into this area so that your hands are pushed up by your stomach. Once you connect to this area, put a hand next to you and lift the legs so that you have a 90-degree angle in your hips and knees. Keep the feet together. Next, move the knees a bit farther forward so that you engage your abdominal muscles but do not lose contact between your lower back and the floor. Breathe in and try to push air into your pelvis so that it expands. On the subsequent inhale, contract the pelvic floor muscles by using the same muscles you would to interrupt the flow of urine.

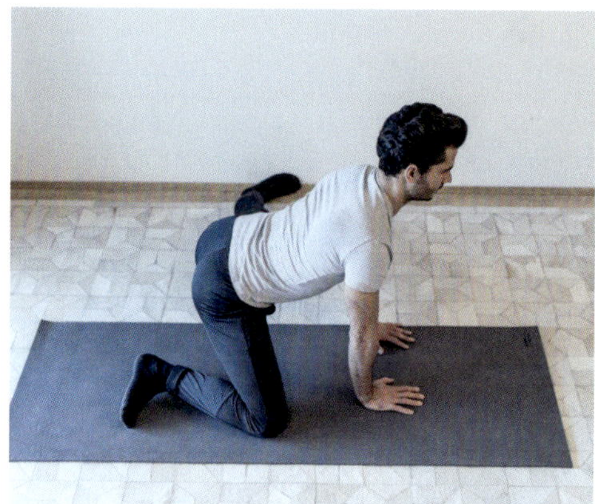
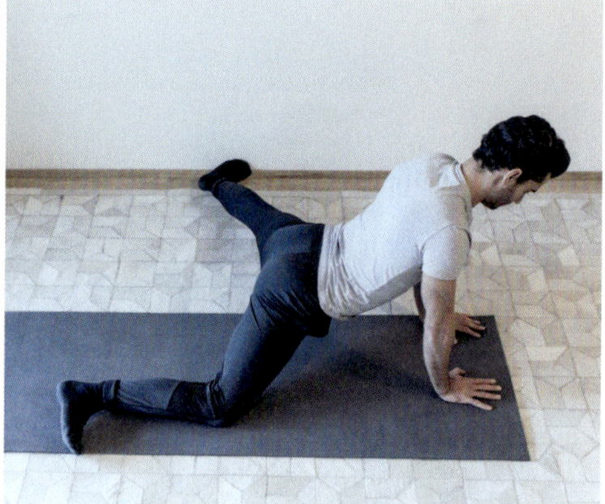

Fig. 3.66: Single-leg wall split (hold for 5 breaths)

Start on all fours next to a wall. Stretch one leg out to the side so that the foot is against the wall. Rock back and forth slowly, feeling a stretch in your inner thighs, moving the sensation of the stretch from the back hip to the front hip. When you rock back, try to keep the arch in your lower back as much as possible, and when you rock forward, engage your core muscles to prevent the lower back from arching too much. Stay in each position for 5 breaths.

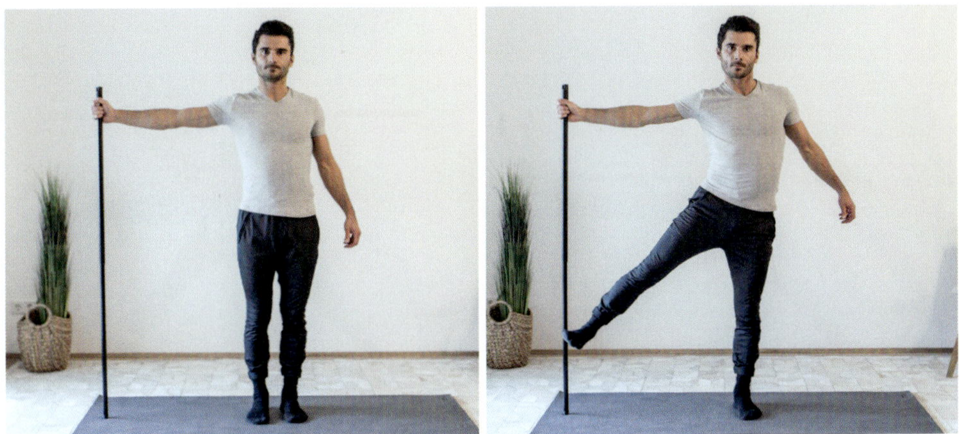

Fig. 3.67: Standing hip abduction with stick (hold 2 x for 5 breaths)

Stand upright, holding the stick next to you with the arm outstretched. Press the stick gently into the floor and move the same side's foot toward the stick until the heel touches it, keeping the leg straight throughout the movement. Push the foot against the stick, engaging the outer hip muscles.

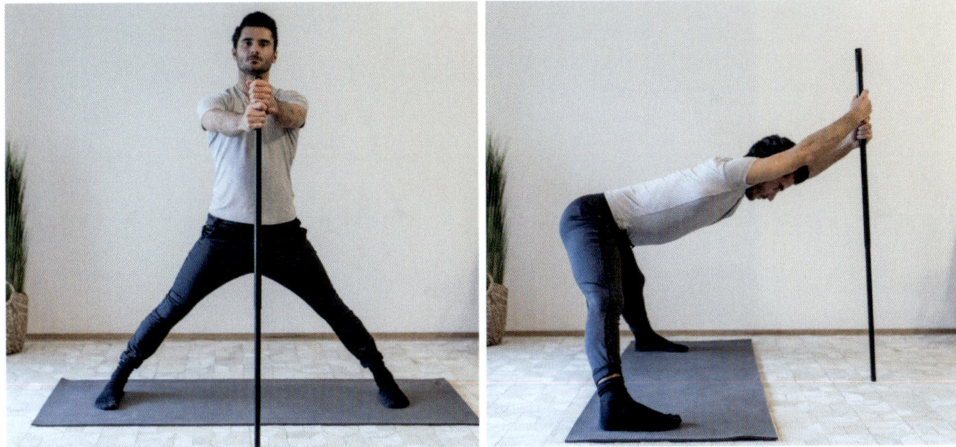

Fig. 3.68: Split with stick (hold for 10 breaths)

Get into the widest split position possible and then bring your feet a bit closer together again. Stretch your arms out in front of you and then hinge forward, pushing the stick gently into the floor. Lower your upper body to the point where you can still maintain a straight spine. Focus on pushing the hips back and the stick forward to elongate your spine.

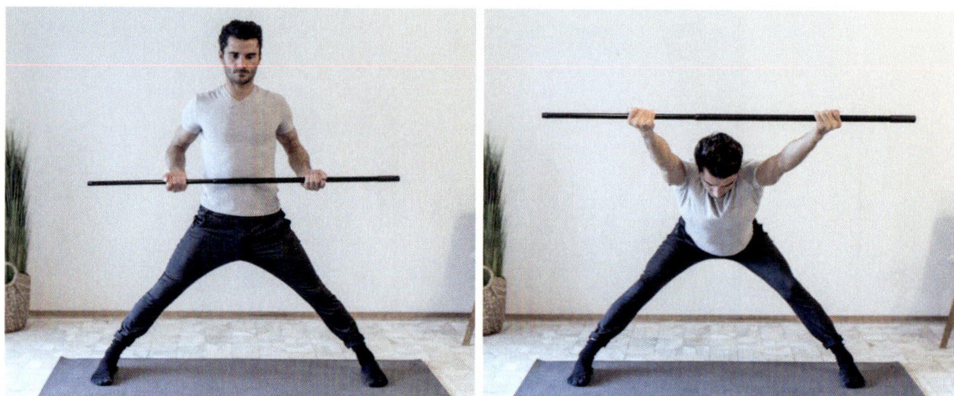

Fig. 3.69: Split with stick raised (hold for 10 breaths)

Get into the widest split position possible and then bring your feet a bit closer together again. Hold the stick at your stomach with your hands a bit wider than shoulder-width apart and facing up. Bringing the stick forward, lower your upper body to the point where you can maintain a straight spine. Bend the knees slightly and keep the arms aligned with the spine. Stay in this position. Breathe three-dimensionally and focus on pushing the hips back and the stick forward to elongate your spine.

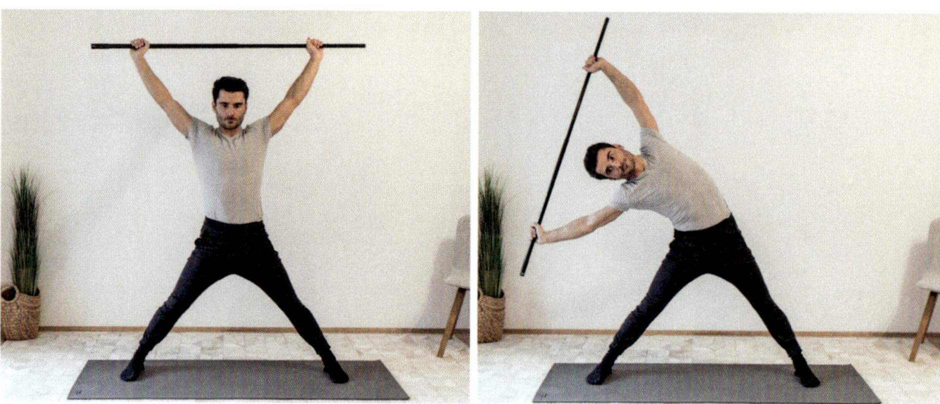

Fig. 3.70: Split with side bend (hold for 10 breaths)

Get into the widest split position possible and then bring your feet a bit closer together again. Hold the stick above your head with the hands a bit wider than shoulder-width and facing forward. Bend over to one side as far as you can while the lower hand is pulling the stick down and the upper hand is pushing the stick forward and up. Keep your knees bent slightly and your arms aligned with your spine.

Cool-Down

After every training session, no matter how long it was, do the following breathing exercise to bring balance back into your breathing and nervous system.

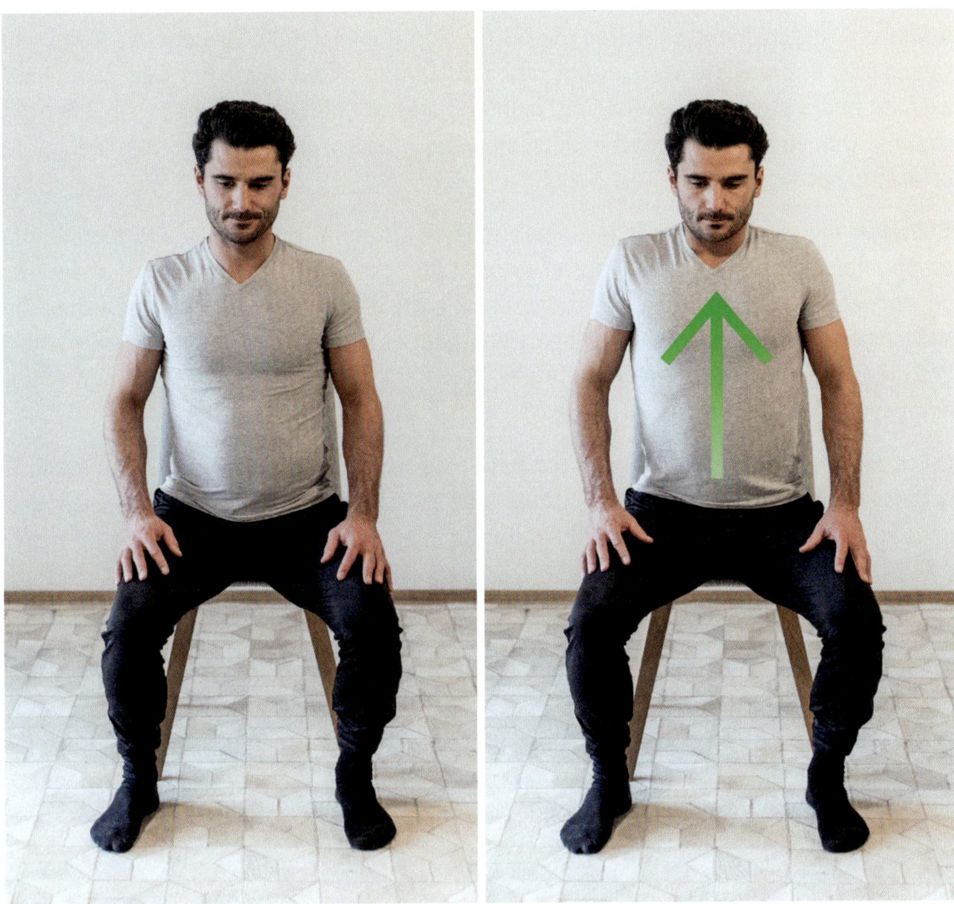

Fig. 3.71: Balanced breathing (5 circles)

Sit on a chair with your spine in a neutral position and your hands on your lap. Breathe in slowly, filling your stomach first; let the air then move up to your rib cage, and finally use the neck to draw in the last bits of air. This inhalation phase should take 5 seconds. Next, hold your breath for another 5 seconds and then exhale slowly again for 5 seconds, while your stomach and chest come down again. Hold for 5 seconds before taking the next breath. It is important that you breathe slowly and consciously and do not force inhalation or exhalation. Once the 5-second cycle becomes easy, you can try to extend every phase to 6 seconds, then 7 seconds, and so on.

TWEAKING THE PLAN

If certain exercises in your training plan are too difficult or actually cause pain, don't push through them. Your structures might still be too sensitive for it, or you've lost optimal form after the first few repetitions. Instead think of how you could tweak the exercise to make it less uncomfortable for you or just skip it completely. This doesn't mean you should stop any exercise once it gets hard, but learn to differentiate between just a hard exercise and a structure-overloading, painful one. For example, your neck shouldn't get so tense that you get a headache. Remember, neck tension often comes from inefficient breathing patterns.

To tweak the exercises, lower the repetitions or duration, slow down and focus more on optimal form, or just use whatever support you can think of in order to make it less uncomfortable for you. The final exercises of each of the five parts can be especially challenging. Don't worry if you can't perform them as required yet; with patience you will get there. Training more gently might just be what your body needs at the moment to empty your barrel.

On the flipside, if the exercises are too easy for you, and you don't feel like anything is actually happening in your body, think of ways to make them harder. Use a greater arm lever, add some weight, or extend the duration in order to challenge yourself a bit more.

MY APPRAISAL

This section is particularly suitable for you if you have recurring back problems and know that you won't be able to pass at least three out of the five tests. In this case, the exercises will help you put out your match so that the problems don't reappear as soon as your barrel is a little fuller again. They're also relevant if you do a lot of sports or go to the gym regularly because then your quality of movement is even more important. In these cases, select a higher number for the first question about your conviction.

Your action steps:

1. **Do the self-tests and choose the exercises accordingly.**

→ Do all of the five self-tests, and if you don't pass many of them and there will be too many exercises in your plan, you can also split the plan and do half of the exercises on one day and the other half the next day.

2. **Try the exercises out.**

→ Perform the exercises and note what works for you and what doesn't.

3. **Tweak the plan and train regularly.**

→ Change whatever you need to change and challenge yourself to do the exercises as often as possible.

How convinced are you that the action steps in this area can help you?
On a scale of 1-10:

0	1	2	3	4	5	6	7	8	9	10

How much do the action steps inspire you; do you feel like doing them?
On a scale of 1-10:

0	1	2	3	4	5	6	7	8	9	10

How likely are you to implement the action steps?
On a scale of 1-10:

0	1	2	3	4	5	6	7	8	9	10

EFFORTLESS

3.3.2 FAVORITE ACTIVITIES

In the previous section, we learned how important movement is for us and how well it empties the barrel. Nevertheless, most people nowadays move far too little. People who have back problems, in particular, often still think that they need to be very careful with their back and consequently may move even less often.

Though this is a natural reaction to acute pain, permanently moving less only makes the pain worse. So, after the initial pain has subsided, it makes sense to return directly to your usual daily activities and try to move as much and as normally as possible.

When we feel restricted because of our pain, we think we need to take it easy on ourselves and no longer engage in the activities that we like, that we're used to doing, and that mean a lot to us. This can bring us down and cause enormous distress. It leads us into a vicious circle of worry, fear, immobility, and lasting pain.

If, however, we manage to remain active as usual and pursue our favorite activities, we can quickly get out of this vicious circle. While exercise in general is already very beneficial, it's the meaning and fun of certain activities that greatly increases the positive effects of an activity.

Exercising simply because you "should" exercise, for example in the gym or in rehabilitation sports, might not be as beneficial as pursuing the activities that you personally prefer to do. These activities are is as individual as a fingerprint. For some, it's playing with their grandchildren, for others it's walking outdoors or going to their favorite Yoga class, and for others it's just doing their favorite sport.

We can't remedy all of the stress and tension we accumulate from sitting all day by going to the gym once a week, but if we get back to doing our favorite activities on a regular basis, even in between phases of long sitting, we increase the chances of giving our body a sufficient amount of movement regularly to make up for it.

For me, my favorite activity has always been playing soccer. Even after my injury I found a way to keep on playing, and even though I wasn't as fit as I used to be, I still had a lot of fun and fulfillment playing it again.

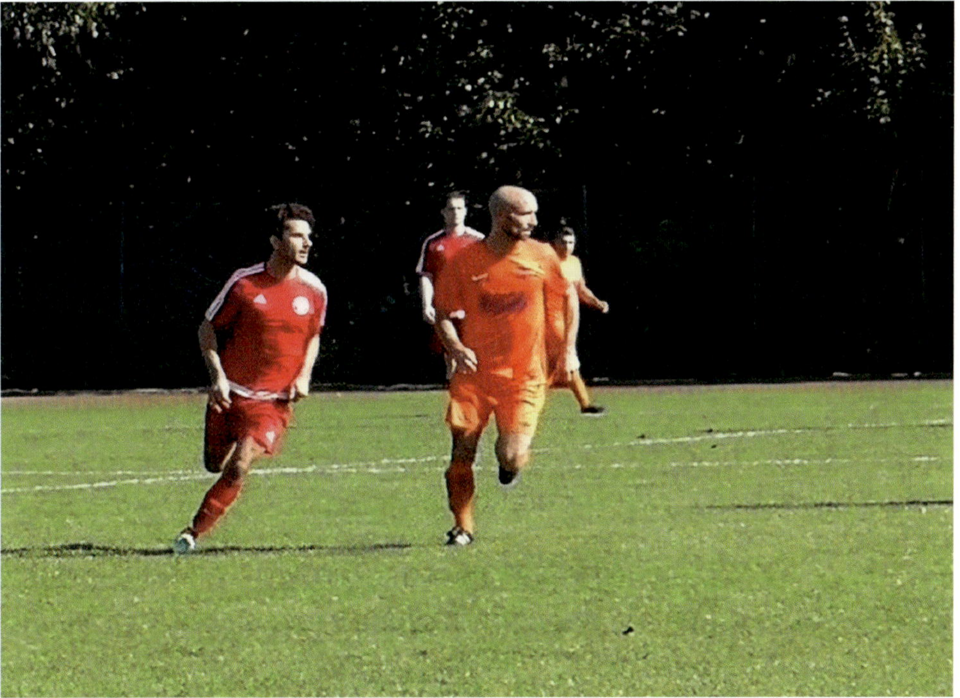

Fig. 3.72: When doing our favorite activity, we might be able to do more than we thought we could. After I hadn't even been jogging for years, I was able to run, jump, twist, and kick the ball again.

We're often unaware of the movements that are really fun, inspiring, and meaningful to us. Many people believe they are just too lazy to move in general whereas the movements they think they have to do simply don't appeal to them. Going to the gym costs so much effort that most people's motivation only lasts a few weeks, and then they pay the fees month after month without even seeing the inside of the gym again.

Is it really due to our sedentary way of life, or is it that many people find exercises on the machines too boring? They feel like running on a treadmill is like running in a hamster wheel, or some simply feel overwhelmed in group classes.

But when we think back, every person finds at least one sport or physical activity that he or she liked doing. For some it was playing soccer with their friends, for others dancing outdoors, and for the mother it was playing around with her children.

Whatever activity we enjoy, it makes sense to reintegrate it into our daily lives. In many cases, it's even necessary to have a fully functional and painless body, and if our body knows it has something to be fit and pain free for, then it's more likely to actually become fit again.

But we often forget what it was, or we don't see ourselves doing that again because perhaps we think our injury hinders us, we're too old, or we wouldn't find anyone to join us.

For a while I believed that fitness training was my favorite activity, and it completely replaced soccer. I thought to myself: Since I can't or shouldn't practice it anymore anyway, I don't want to have anything to do with it. Only when I gave myself permission to believe that I could play again at some point did I rediscover my love for this sport.

By using the following questions, we can try to find out what your favorite activities are. Simply answer each question and enter the activities or sports that occur most frequently under "Result."

DETERMINE YOUR FAVORITE ACTIVITIES

1. What are your favorite activities or sports? Or what activity would be inspiring for you to be able to do?

   Answer:

   ____

   ____

2. What activities or sports were you able to do for hours without stopping?

   Answer:

   ____

   ____

3. What activities or sports would you like to do again if you had a pain-free and fit body? Or what ones are you afraid of doing because of your symptoms?

   Answer:

   ____

   ____

Now select the activity or sport that occurred most often. This activity is the best one to engage in to empty your barrel.

Result:

____

____

Additional question: If your pain is very restrictive, what are individual movements or postures that you would like to be able to perform or take up again without problems? For example, bending over, twisting the spine, jumping, sitting on the floor, kneeling.

Answer:

____

____

PREPARING FOR THE ACTIVITY

As a warm-up, it's beneficial to get your hips and thoracic spine more mobile to take compensatory stress away from the back. So as a preparation you can do your specific exercises from section 3.2.1 in case you found some potential for improvement.

Think about what a good intensity and duration would be to start with and progress from there. Also consider the environment you want to do the activity in. It should be one that's inspiring and that doesn't cause much stress. As recent studies have shown, our stress levels can be lowered in the great outdoors in the fresh air where we feel freer. Therefore, hiking or jogging in the forest is especially recommended when the full barrel is creating a lot of distress.

Also, you might consider doing sports with friends who will make it more fun, listening to your favorite music to move more joyfully, or withdrawing away from all the stress of everyday life to a quiet place.

If you have certain movements (additional question from the questionnaire) that you no longer feel able to perform, think about the following. During your favorite activity, you may be noticing how complexly you're able to move again and how long your body can withstand stress. Then why not this single movement as well? Have the courage to approach doing it again, perhaps first using a wall or something similar as a support, but remain fearless as best you can.

MY APPRAISAL

This area is especially suitable for you if you aren't pursuing your favorite activity/ sport because you're afraid that it could aggravate your symptoms, or if you move cautiously in everyday motions. Also if you generally don't move much or if you prefer to do activities that are fun and inspiring instead of following a prescribed exercise program. In these cases, select a higher number for the first question about your conviction.

Your action steps:

1. **Find your favorite activity.**

→ Do the "Determine Your Favorite Activities" questionnaire and pick the activity you list most often.

2. **Prepare it.**

→ Plan your approach and maybe find someone to do it with you.

3. **Warm up and be brave enough to do it.**

→ Use the individual exercises from chapter 3.1 for a warm-up. Also, in the upcoming weeks, make sure you increase the duration of your favorite activity by as many minutes as you think would be effortlessly possible.

How convinced are you that the action steps in this area can help you?
On a scale of 1-10:

0	1	2	3	4	5	6	7	8	9	10

How inspired are you by the action steps?
On a scale of 1-10:

0	1	2	3	4	5	6	7	8	9	10

How likely are you to implement the action steps?
On a scale of 1-10:

0	1	2	3	4	5	6	7	8	9	10

E F F O R T L E S S

3.3.3 FUEL

Just like gasoline is necessary to fuel a car, food is necessary to fuel our lives. Even more than just fuel, food is also a building material. Carbohydrates and fats provide us with energy; protein and water are responsible for building cells and tissue; and vitamins and minerals form enzymes and regulate the metabolism. Without doubt, our food is the best medicine nature has to offer us.

If we internalize the following basic idea, "eating to live instead of living to eat," we're well on our way to taking advantage of food and emptying our barrel. This doesn't mean that we shouldn't enjoy and celebrate food anymore, but rather it's more about internalizing this basic attitude to automatically make the right decisions concerning food and taking away any stress that more and more people impose on themselves in order not to eat anything "bad."

Because with all the different diets and nutritional philosophies coming at us from all sides, be it veganism, paleo, or ketogenic diet, one form of nutrition has proven over the years to be the most reasonable, sustainable, and simplest: the "normal one." This doesn't necessarily mean the diet of most people in the western world, but simply the varied, moderate, and, above all, regular diet.

In this well-balanced diet, no food is necessarily "forbidden" (excepting food intolerances or allergies), but also no food is praised as a miraculous "superfood." The goal is to eat a variety of food, preferably nutritious foods, while being moderate with the consumption of desserts, snacks, processed foods, and so on. All forms of nutrition have advantages and disadvantages in the short or long term and certain foods can be exactly right for some people but problematic for others. By following rigid fad diets and placing strong judgment on the food we eat, we take away our own sense of knowing what's good for us and what can potentially cause inner conflict.

Food should be simple, and there is no need to stress out by counting calories all the time, having to read every ingredient on the label, or weighing everything with a scale (unless you like to do so or have a specific performance goal). So, we can instead make it easy by following simple guidelines when putting together portions for our meals. These guidelines are as follows:

FOOD COMPOSITION FORMULATION

- The size of your fist determines the amount of vegetables or fruit you eat.
- Your palm determines the amount of protein (e.g., meat, cheese, or soy).
- Your palm determines the amount of carbohydrates (though this serving can be slightly larger than your palm).
- The volume of your thumb determines the portion of fat-dense foods.

It's recommended that men eat two portions of each type of food per meal, and women, one portion. These guidelines are for those who eat three to four times a day. While these are of course only very rough recommendations, and it always depends on the physical proportions of the individual person, they make healthy nutrition simple and stress free.

Another way to eat a "normal" diet is to follow the recommendations for nutrition as outlined by the Harvard Medical School (2011). The plate shows how much of each food should make up a well-balanced meal. Vegetables make up the largest part, proteins from meat, fish, or dairy products as well as carbohydrates, preferably from whole grains, each make up a quarter, whereas the fruit and vegetable portion makes up half. In general, whole and regional foods should be used whenever possible.

50% FRUITS AND VEGETABLES
25% PROTEIN-RICH FOODS
25% FIBER-RICH CARBOHYDRATES

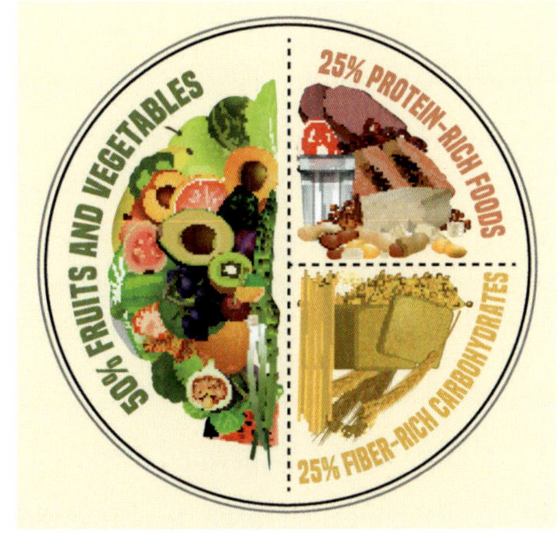

Fig. 3.73: Food plate, showing the Harvard Medical School nutrition recommendation (2011)

How well are you following these guidelines? Is there an area you already know you struggle with? Or is there an area where you commonly exceed these recommendations?

Not included in this plate is the recommendation for the intake of liquids. Only if we consume enough liquids can our tissues be optimally supplied with nutrients and waste or toxins be eliminated. Drinking at least half a gallon (2 liters) of fluid per day is indispensable in order to stop joint problems. Though, drinking enough liquids doesn't mean upping your coffee, alcohol, or sweetened beverage consumption. Those should be consumed in moderation only, and water should make up the biggest part of your daily fluid intake.

Anti-inflammatory diet

As described in section 2.2.7, inflammatory foods can cause inflammatory processes in our body. Fortunately, there are also numerous foods that can counteract inflammation. If we increasingly integrate these into our diet, this can put a stop to the inflammatory processes.

Following you'll find a list of a variety of inflammatory and anti-inflammatory foods. In addition, dietary supplements are also listed because, for example, the additional intake of vitamin D3 can be particularly useful in winter. The lack of sunlight during the winter leads to the weakening of bones and muscle functions and can also contribute to filling the barrel, and additional vitamin D3 can counteract this. However, dietary supplements should never be taken as a substitute for a healthy diet. A professional consultation about which dietary supplements make the most sense in an individual case is certainly helpful.

Inflammatory foods

- All refined wheat products (gluten), pasta, cereals, pretzels, crackers, desserts, and all other foods made from cereals or flour.
- Hardened fats (trans fats), which are found in margarine, fried foods, and most packaged, readymade meals as well as in corn oil, thistle oil, sunflower oil, soybean oil, mayonnaise, and yogurt dressing.
- Lemonades and sugar.
- Milk or soy products when used as a staple food.
- Eggs from caged rather than free-range chickens.
- Omega-6 fatty acids and flavor enhancers such as glutamic acid (glutamate).

Anti-inflammatory foods

- All fruits and vegetables (preferably raw or steamed).
- Sweet potatoes.
- Wild salmon, mackerel, and sardines.
- Red meat, poultry, and eggs from grass-fed animals; omega-3 eggs.
- Nuts: raw almonds, cashew nuts, walnuts, hazelnuts, macadamia nuts, etc. (but not too many, as they contain many calories).
- Spices, such as ginger, turmeric, frankincense, garlic, oregano, paprika, cayenne pepper, rosemary, coriander, seaweed, basil, sea salt, Himalayan salt.
- Pasture butter, ghee, extra-virgin olive oil, balsamic vinegar, mustard.
- Water or tea and, in moderation, red wine.
- Dark chocolate.
- Food supplements: omega-3 fatty acids (best from krill oil), vegetable multivitamin preparation, and vitamin D3.

Which of these anti-inflammatory foods are you inspired to eat more? When prepared well, you might be surprised how good they can taste. There are several websites that give recipes which include mainly anti-inflammatory food.

But we don't have to try eating a completely anti-inflammatory diet right away. Adding in small amounts of anti-inflammatory foods to our diets have a more long-term effect than radical changes, which are usually not sustained in the long term and then trigger the well-known yo-yo effect. Though, this shouldn't stop you from following a particular detox program if perhaps you had success with it in the past, and it's something you are inspired to do again.

Eating behavior

Having a better colon peristalsis and aligning food intake with the body's daily rhythms (circadian rhythms), meal timing, and a more balanced mental attitude toward our diet can help just as much as some other healthy eating behaviors, which, though still highly relevant, are no longer part of everyday practice for most people. Here is a list of those healthy behaviors:

TIPS FOR HEALTHY EATING BEHAVIOUR

- No large meals for four hours before going to bed.
- Avoid "overeating."
- Rest and eat consciously.
- Eat regularly (preferably three or even up to five times a day), but no snacking.
- Vary your food, but do not mix too much at once.
- Eat in an upright sitting position.
- Be grateful for your food and don't feel bad after eating something not so healthy.
- Never eat burned foods as the acrylamide produced can have toxic effects on your body.
- Nap before rather than after eating and instead take a digestive walk afterwards.
- Chew food well.

Action steps:

1. **Pick one big thing and change it.**

→ What is the one thing that you think you're lacking the most but that you actually can change pretty effortlessly? Eating more protein? Drinking more water? Eating breakfast? Ditching the soda? Pick one thing and change it in your everyday life.

2. **Exchange one inflammatory food with one anti-inflammatory food.**

→ What is the one food you can easily swap? And what could be an inspiring food to eat more often? Pick one from each side and replace them.

3. **Change one behavior.**

→ Is there a behavior around eating that you could change effortlessly? Maybe it even goes hand in hand with a big thing from action step 1, such as eating breakfast and not eating late at night. Pick one behavior you will focus on changing.

MY APPRAISAL

This area is especially appropriate for you if your gastrointestinal tract often causes problems, you have little energy in your everyday life, or you know that you generally eat a rather unhealthy diet. In these cases, select a higher number for the first question about your conviction.

How convinced are you that the action steps in this area can help you?
On a scale of 1-10:

0	1	2	3	4	5	6	7	8	9	10

How much do the action steps inspire you; how much do you feel like doing them?
On a scale of 1-10:

0	1	2	3	4	5	6	7	8	9	10

How likely are you to implement the action steps?
On a scale of 1-10:

0	1	2	3	4	5	6	7	8	9	10

E F F O R T L E S S

3.3.4 OPTIMIZING THE ENVIRONMENT

So far, we've learned what we can do to change our own internal environment, but bringing about changes in the external environment might be just as beneficial for our long-term back health. For the environments in which we live and work, we have to determine how well each facilitates movement and supports our regeneration—all factors that can increase the chances of emptying the barrel. Plus, they also have a great influence on our genetic expression (those genes that are used to create the proteins in our body), as we learned in the first chapter about epigenetics.

So now we want to look at your environment and find the small things we can change in your everyday life to empty your barrel. These changes can be very simple, for example, the clothes and shoes you wear—perhaps they're too tight—backpacks or other bags you carry everywhere, or even bras that don't let you breathe from the diaphragm. Are there any other changes you can make that you know will promote back health?

What's important is that even when you can't change certain things in your environment, you don't make those circumstances responsible for your pain and fall into the victim role, but rather see where there is actual potential for improvement and actively approach changing the circumstances you're able to change.

Movement at our workplace is particularly important in order to get in the 10,000 steps we're supposed to take every day. For that, you can try to increase the aforementioned NEAT activities, especially if you're working in a sedentary job. There are small changes you can make at work so that you must move more. For example, you could deliberately park your car farther from your office building, or you can even leave the car at home and walk to work. In the office you can place the printer far away from you so that you must get up and walk a bit every time you need to use it. If you decide to not use the telephone to communicate with your colleagues anymore, it will encourage you to take those few steps to get the info you need from them in person.

Each static (motion-free) phase should always be alternated with motion. If you do so, then slouching for a while, a forward head posture, or an arched back position is totally fine because regular movement can dampen their negative effects.

Because generally it's unfavorable to maintain one position over a longer period of time, it's important to add regular exercise every day. The recommendation for office workers is to move at least once an hour for about five minutes. This can counteract muscle and fascia shortening, increase productivity, and help prevent the possibility of other diseases which result from a sedentary lifestyle. You can move by doing stretching exercises, going outside for a breath of fresh air, or taking a little walk, for example.

The old way to change the working environment to encourage more activity was by sticking reminder notes on the computer screen, but more often than not, you stop noticing them after two weeks at the latest. So nowadays there are many apps that remind you to move, or simply setting an alarm for every hour would be an option, too.

Removing obstacles that hinder activity in everyday life

Oftentimes, there are circumstances that prevent us from doing our favorite activities, or activities in general. Perhaps our bicycle is broken, we need new running shoes, or we moved and our favorite gym isn't around the corner anymore. Instead of giving in to these excuses, we can acknowledge them and change our circumstances. We could go and buy a new bicycle or new running shoes or just look for another gym close by.

The new membership in a gym could be a first impulse for doing regular exercise again. Finding a training partner would then increase the motivation because of the commitment we make with the other person, and it just might be more fun to go there together. Thinking about what it is in our external circumstances that prevent us from doing certain activities and what we could do to adjust them will enable us to remove those obstacles.

Creating a regeneration-friendly environment

We need a regeneration-friendly environment, especially for sleeping because while sleeping our body functions are reduced, muscle tone as well as blood pressure and heart rate decrease, we breathe more slowly, and our body temperature also decreases slightly.

After all the efforts of the day, our body and especially the brain can optimally recover. Damage to the organism is now repaired, and cells are renewed.

However, if sleep deprivation occurs, or if we don't have a good night's sleep, the body lacks this opportunity to recover well. The consequences are reduced performance, poor concentration, and increased susceptibility to stress. Disturbing our bodies' natural rhythms also causes dysfunctions in our muscle tension, breathing patterns, heartrate, blood pressure, body temperature, hormones, metabolism, and other functions. All of this can fill our barrel to the brim.

In addition to adhering to a sleep rhythm and personal sleep rituals (e.g., counting sheep, meditation, or reading a book), it makes sense to also change the environment in such a way that we can achieve sufficient and restful sleep.

Light plays an important role here, because light in the bedroom inhibits the release of melatonin. Sufficient melatonin is needed to make us tired. If our body produces too little because it receives the signal from all the light that it's daytime, we're more likely to stay in a state of wakefulness. So, the bedroom should be completely dark. If that's not possible, we can put on a sleep mask.

The release of melatonin is also inhibited by the blue light from mobile phones, televisions, or computers. We shouldn't expose ourselves to any more blue light at least one hour before going to bed. There are also good blue light filter apps that filter the light to prevent this mechanism from working. Blue light filter glasses would also be an option if we wanted to work on the computer late in the evening.

During the day, however, we need the blue light to be able to produce the "happiness hormone" serotonin. This ensures that we're awake and in a good mood, and it can also inhibit pain. Due to the interaction of these two hormones, the more serotonin our body releases during the day, the more melatonin our body can release in the evening. Since we don't get enough sunlight in the winter months, we should use more artificial light sources during the day so that we can fall asleep more easily at night.

Disturbing noises can also prevent us from getting a good night's sleep. If the complete elimination of noise isn't possible, earplugs or devices that drown out the noise with white noise can be used. There are also specific apps that can do this.

The temperature in the bedroom also plays an important role. It should be comfortable, but not too high, 65-70 °F (18-20 °C) is optimal.

Lastly, having a bed system that is optimally tailored to your needs and has a mattress that promotes the neutral position of your spine as well as movement at night helps your spine recover optimally at night, too.

Action Steps:

1. **Include more NEAT activities at work.**

→ Pick one circumstance in your work environment and change it so that you will have to move more.

2. **Eliminate obstacles and excuses.**

→ Pick one obstacle that hinders your activities and remove it. At least you will have one less excuse then.

3. **Emphasize better regeneration at home.**

→ Pick one circumstance at home and change it, such as making your bedroom darker, so you can recover better.

MY APPRAISAL

This area is especially appropriate for you if you often feel drained and worn out, if you find yourself coming up with lots of excuses for not being more active, or if you don't feel like getting enough or good quality sleep. In these cases, select a higher number for the first question about your conviction.

How convinced are you that the action steps in this area can help you?
On a scale of 1-10:

0	1	2	3	4	5	6	7	8	9	10

How inspired are you to do the action steps?
On a scale of 1-10:

0	1	2	3	4	5	6	7	8	9	10

How likely are you to implement the action steps?
On a scale of 1-10:

0	1	2	3	4	5	6	7	8	9	10

EFFORTLESS

3.3.5 REASON DETERMINATION

When it comes to pain, we often get emotional, and our view of how things really are becomes blurred. We only see the downside of the pain and want to get rid of it as quick as possible. Besides being in fight or flight mode because of that, we also often adopt negative thoughts like: "This is just terrible" or: "I will be suffering for the rest of my life." But as we learned in the second chapter on current pain research, our chances of recovery are enormously influenced by our attitudes toward ourselves, our diagnosis, and our external circumstances. So, our main interest now is to correct ways of thinking such as catastrophic thoughts, excessive generalizations, or striving for perfection. Although those negative thought patterns may be justified because the pain is so severe and the limitations so great, keeping them will activate the nocebo effect which will only fill the barrel up more and more.

If, however, we learn to see a reason behind our pain and get the message the pain wanted to teach us, the symptoms consume less of our thoughts and may even quiet down. Taking on a corresponding belief system can be very empowering and can give us control over our body, keeping the victim mentality at bay. Moreover, this cognitive restructuring changes our thought patterns, attitude, and perception in such a way that our behavior is changed. Although there are plenty of other situations in which cognitive restructuring would be helpful, we can now use it to find meaning in the pain, calming our fight or flight response and emptying our barrels.

By looking for the blessings in disguise, you're able to let go of the belief that it's solely a tragedy, and that "the gods must be against you." For me, my injury was a blessing because not only did it get me out of a pretty stressful situation I was struggling to cope with, but it also gave me the opportunity to live my greatest dream which was to spend a semester abroad in Santa Barbara and visit my favorite places in the world. Moreover, it also pushed me to learn more about my own body and all of the great training methods out there, thereby paving the way for me to my current profession and the desire to write this book.

Asking ourselves the right questions will bring us answers that make us grateful because we will have a better understanding of our pain, will change the way we think about our pain, and we will empty our barrels. Instead of asking "why me?" or "why can't I just have a pain-free life?", we can ask ourselves "what benefits has the pain caused?", "what can I learn from my pain?", or "what doors did it open for me?" If we set our emotional bias aside and try to use more objective reasoning to answer the question, "why do I have this pain," we find the upsides of the pain, lift a lot of negative emotions from our shoulders, and increase the chance that the pain will ease.

But first we need to understand how our brain (i.e., the Pulvinar Nuclei in the Thalamus) filters the information from the environment according to our highest priorities, meaning, the things that are most important to us. When we consider that we subconsciously tend to give high priority to things that are most important to us and organize our lives accordingly, we're more likely to find the benefits in our current state. Only then can we also understand why we might have been given other priorities besides our back health more time and attention in the past.

As an example of those subconscious filters consider a pregnant woman strolling through a shopping mall with her husband, who's a car mechanic by trade. The woman will immediately notice the baby clothes store, though the man didn't notice it at all. Instead, he noticed the car store as soon as he came in. Rather than accompanying his wife to the baby shop, he wants to go to the car shop, because we're intrinsically motivated for things that correspond to our highest priorities.

Because that is how our brains function, we now want to get those subconscious reasons to surface in order to find meaning in the pain, which will lower its amplitude. To do this, first think carefully about the three things in your life that are most important to you. Every person has his or her individual highest priorities. These aren't necessarily what you fantasize about but what your life actually contains because you spend the most time, money, or thoughts on them. They can be your children, career, travelling, reading, fitness, personal development, or spirituality.

After you write down those three priorities, create a list and put down all the benefits to these priorities that your back problems have yielded by asking yourself the following questions:

- How do the back problems help me achieve what's most important?
- What opportunities did the pain bring?
- How did the pain make me the person I am today?
- What did the pain push me to do or to study?

Make sure you include answers from all seven levels of life:

professional

1. financial
2. family
3. physical
4. social
5. mental
6. spiritual

Also, ask yourself the following question in relation to each these seven areas:
How do my back problems help me make progress in this level?

Can you perhaps escape the work stress for a bit and make time for other important things? Do you feel you socialize enough with others? Does it help you to say no to people, now that you have an excuse for it? Or have you been able to learn something about your own body that pushed you to live a healthier life in general?

There are no wrong answers, and there can be many different answers or only a few but very strong and meaningful ones. Even if you don't find the benefits right away, keep on looking. Try to answer the questions until you can really see and feel that you recognized the reason for your pain and that the pain actually comes with equal benefits.

Find reasons for your back health

Of course, after finding all the benefits the pain brought you, you shouldn't just come to terms with having an unhealthy back, as the goal of this book is to encourage you to achieve a sustainable healthy back. For that we need you to have a greater reason to be pain free and to do the necessary action steps that will get you there.

So we must find more advantages than disadvantages of a healthy back, otherwise your current thoughts and resulting actions might not get you there. But when your "Why" has become big enough, the "how" will take care of itself. You really have to know why you want to become healthy again, or it might not happen.

Finding enough benefits of having a sustainable, healthy back will let your "why" grow to the point where it eventually exceeds everything that stops you from creating that healthy back.

So, the following exercise is going to be about finding at least 100 advantages of having a healthy back while also considering secondary or tertiary reasons. For example: If I have less pain, I'm in a better mood, and this has a positive effect on my relationship.

To stimulate your imagination a little, I've listed 20 possible advantages. You're allowed to copy a few of these advantages which apply to you, but you must also find your own; otherwise the exercise won't work.

20 BENEFITS OF HAVING A HEALTHY BACK

1. less pain and tension
2. more flexibility
3. sitting or standing longer without problems
4. good role model for your own children
5. higher performance
6. better mood
7. better organ function
8. regain 2 to 3 cm (1 in.) in body height
9. better posture
10. no longer relying on passive treatments
11. less worry and fear about injuring the back
12. playing with children longer
13. save on medication, rehabilitation, or aids
14. fewer visits to the doctor
15. being able to do sports with friends again
16. better breathing
17. better concentration
18. more productive work
19. better blood circulation
20. being less dependent on others

This activity requires a lot of work, and often after the first 20 to 30 advantages you reach the limits of your imagination. But from that point on, especially, the effects are the greatest. Since the brain is highly malleable, by intensively brooding we create completely new circuits in the brains synapses which can lead to long-term changes in our priorities.

You also want to think of the benefits of learning new things in the process. That would be for example, to learn to persevere with something, to feel proud of yourself for accomplishing something or to learn to do something for yourself instead of mainly sacrificing yourself for others.

Next, try to find advantages of how a healthy back can help you with these priorities. Go through the seven areas of life again and find advantages in each of these areas. Consider, for example, the financial area, and your priority would be your children. One advantage of a healthy back would be that you would be fit enough to do sports with your children instead of having to invite them to the theme park. This helps you on a financial level, because you can save a lot of money.

If the exercise has worked, your behavior should´ve changed and you´re more likely to make decisions that help your back health. If not, then work on finding more benefits and try to feel them for real, rather than just quickly adding something abstract or unclear ones to get done.

Visualize your reasons

After you've realized that your problems also bring benefits and your "why" for performing your back-health plan has developed, creating a vision of what your life will look like with a healthy back, more quality of life, and increased performance further motivates you by giving you a clear mental picture of your goals for the future. That sharpens your awareness to filter out the things that will get you there.

So, this exercise is about identifying your reasons for sustained back health and visualizing your reasons as part of a realistic plan.

Visualizing that future free of back pain more clearly will give you greater inner motivation and vitality, and as a result, you will be more likely to realize it.

Only when I started to imagine exactly what it would mean if I could play soccer again without any problems did I slowly but surely start to make it a reality. If we don't have a clear goal in mind, then we won't know where the journey should take us; we will end up stalling.

Answer the following questions to form a clear vision:

1. What would your optimal day look like if your back was completely healthy, and you were just bursting with vitality?
2. What would your complete daily routine be, from getting up to going to bed?
3. What exactly are your goals with regard to your back health?

4. With regard to playing with the kids?
5. With regard to playing sports with your friends?
6. With regard to dancing?

You want to make sure that you stay realistic, though. Since the body is extremely plastic, there have been cases of unbelievable recoveries in the past, but there must be reasonable timeframes and enough focused activities achieve recovery. When I changed from practicing soccer two times a week to six times a week, my body reacted, and I suffered inflamed Achilles tendons. So even if it takes longer than you wanted, keep that vision in mind and persevere. Whenever you get stuck and feel like you've hit some roadblocks, focus on your vision again, and you'll overcome the obstacle and get your energy back.

Actually, having the vision in front of you helps to keep your focus. So create a vision board with pictures and hang it up in the bedroom as your daily reminder. You can fill it with pictures of you doing your favorite sport, of you dancing, or of you doing anything else you enjoyed before your back pain. Keeping a visual reminder of your goals will keep you less distracted and focused on the big picture.

Action steps:

1. **Find the reason behind your pain.**

→ Do the exercise to find the gains of your pains. Describe what the benefits and opportunities that your pain has created are. What are the blessings in disguise?

2. **Find the reasons for your back health.**

→ Do the exercise to connect your highest priorities to your back health in order to increase your inner motivation and your "why."

3. **Visualize your reasons.**

→ Find your vision, create a vision board, and work daily on getting into your mind as clearly as possible.

MY APPRAISAL

This area is especially appropriate for you if you have chronic or episodic back problems which you consider to be very bad and have increased your worry and anxiety. Also, if you know that you generally struggling with improving your back health or you are frequently unable to keep up with an activity. In these cases, select a higher number for the first question about your conviction.

How convinced are you that the action steps in this area can help you?
On a scale of 1-10:

0	1	2	3	4	5	6	7	8	9	10

How inspired are you to do the action steps?
On a scale of 1-10:

0	1	2	3	4	5	6	7	8	9	10

How likely are you to implement the action steps?
On a scale of 1-10:

0	1	2	3	4	5	6	7	8	9	10

E F F O R T L E S S

3.3.6 TREATMENTS

A justified approach to remedy back pain is to seek treatment. Today we have access to an incredible variety of healing methods that can eliminate symptoms and greatly alleviate discomfort. These healing methods include medication, manual therapy, massages, operations, chiropractic, osteopathy, acupuncture, cupping, electrotherapy, magnetic field therapy, TCM, dry needling, heat or cold applications, operations, homeopathy, naturopathy, and many other spiritual healing methods. They can do amazing things for your body. A chiropractor can align your spine again and harmonize its discrepancies; a good massage therapist can release the back pain causing sticking points everywhere in the body; and an acupuncturist can manipulate the fascia in a way that it brings balance back into the body. There are so many methods that we can't compare all the advantages and disadvantages in this book, so instead I encourage you to analyze critically which method would be suitable for you and how you could follow it up with appropriate activities. Only relying on passive treatments robs us from having accountability, dignity, and self-worth, and we can become dependent on them.

In order to find suitable treatments for you, you can search for them on the internet or speak to a medical professional. You can also ask yourself a few different questions:

1. Which treatments have helped you in the past?
2. Which treatments have you been recommended by people you trust?
3. Which treatments did you always want to try?

Treatment benefits and risks

In order to increase the chances of getting a good result, you can invest some time in researching the methods you're most interested in and finding objective statistics about their healing possibilities.

Also make sure you're aware of the possible risks before you undergo any treatment. The more educated you are about the benefits and risks of the treatment, the more empowered are you in your decision making. In times of information overload on the internet, it might make sense to ask a specific practitioner for sources of information about the treatment instead of possibly getting misinformed by dubious sources.

Also get informed about what exactly they will do and what it will feel like, instead of just going there and being surprised by what actually happens—like realizing that being poked in the skin with little needles actually hurts. Last but not least, you also want to consider the price, accessibility, and effort you need to put in for the treatment to be effective.

Finding compatible activities

Many people like to give up the responsibility for their back health and rely exclusively on passive healing methods.

Passive healing methods are mostly only really useful for our long-term back health, if we use them in addition to an active lifestyle. If we have an episode of severe, acute back pain behind us, passive methods will support us in becoming active again. If, for example, we take medication after a lumbago to alleviate pain and to reduce the inflammation, it can help us to return to our everyday activities without major restrictions and remain active. But if we use them without this intention, we do nothing to ensure that our barrel is actually being emptied.

We also want to lower the intake as soon as we're getting better so that we don't develop a dependency. If we do not stop taking medication after a few days or weeks, our body begins to reduce the production of its own painkillers (opioids). However, these are important in order to activate the descending inhibition described in section 2.3.1 and desensitize the problem area so that it does not emit pain signals with every small irritation. In addition to the general danger of drugs' side effects, the reduced pain threshold means that the long-term intake of drugs is of particular concern.

However, many people find it so difficult to stop taking their medication because it's the only way for them to get rid of the pain. In order to escape from this vicious circle, it is necessary to learn active methods that help to desensitize the problem area and alleviate pain. The aim of this book is to make us as independent as possible from passive methods by learning how to empty our barrel using active methods without spending a lot of money and time on it as well as living with the possible side effects.

If you want to make sure you do the right activity for your specific problem, ask your practitioner for recommendations on what to do specifically.

Action steps:

1. **Search for suitable treatments.**

→ Make a list of treatments you find on the internet, treatments that have helped you in the past, treatments that have been recommended to you, and treatments that you're interested in.

2. **Research each treatment and select one.**

→ Do the research to find out about healing opportunities and possible risks. Then decide which one you want to try.

3. **Ask for activity recommendations.**

→ Ask your practitioner to recommend activities or exercises that he or she believes would be best in your specific case. Add them to your back-health plan if you're convinced they would help you.

MY APPRAISAL

This area is especially appropriate for you if you feel you need external help with your specific problem, if you generally trust practitioners, or if you are uncertain about the causes of your pain and want an expert to look at it. In these cases, select a higher number for the first question about your conviction.

How convinced are you that the action steps in this area can help you?
On a scale of 1-10:

0	1	2	3	4	5	6	7	8	9	10

How inspired are you to do the action steps?
On a scale of 1-10:

0	1	2	3	4	5	6	7	8	9	10

How likely are you to implement the action steps?
On a scale of 1-10:

0	1	2	3	4	5	6	7	8	9	10

EFFORTLESS

3.3.7 LOAD MANAGEMENT

When it comes to being physically active, people often exhibit two different types of mental attitudes. One attitude is that people believe the more we do, the better it is for us, and then there are those people who believe that if they do nothing at all, they can at least do nothing wrong.

Both attitudes seem to be incorrect when we consider load management theories. Though the disadvantages of insufficient movement have already been discussed a lot in this book, it wasn't meant to promote a "the more, the better" attitude either. If we make changes that are too extreme or we make them too quickly, our bodies won't have enough time to adapt, eventually leading to more pain or even new injuries.

Only when we find the "sweat spot" between those two opposing attitudes do we have optimal development of our fitness and health. In order to maximally improve, all our body structures need an optimal stimulation based on our current fitness level paired with the optimal amount of recovery time. In principle, if the load exceeds our load-bearing capacity, we will overload our system. Physically that can happen when we expose ourselves to an excessive amplitude of load, if the duration of that exposure is too long, or if the exposure is being repeated too often. We commonly fall victim to at least one of those mechanisms when we participate in that yoga or a back fit class that our bodies aren't yet ready for, or when we just can't stop ourselves before we feel completely worn out from our workout.

So it's mandatory to know your current level of fitness before approaching any type of activity. In that regard, it's important to accept that after a phase of acute back pain, our fitness levels might be much lower than before the pain. Walking for just a few minutes can, in the beginning, be the only load that the highly sensitized body structures can bear. So before thinking your body has to be able to bear that load again, think about a reasonable workload that it is actually capable of bearing in that moment.

Soon after I experienced my two herniated discs, I started to train with barbells again because I thought the effects on the muscles would be greater, and I was actually strong enough to exercise with them. What I didn't consider, though, was that my spine was still in an overly sensitized state, and any additional weight was going to irritate it too much. So even though while doing the exercises I didn't feel any pain, when I woke up the next morning, I often felt the pain even more. It wasn't because I didn't sleep well, but because I overloaded my spine the day before.

It's key to objectively look at your current fitness level and approach any type of activity in a logical and patient way. Only then can you empty the barrel optimally by doing your activities.

Ask yourself the following questions:

1. Am I overloading my system and should decrease my load?
2. Am I doing too little and could challenge myself a bit more?

TWEAKING ACTIVITIES

It's important to understand that a high workload doesn't necessarily mean that it comes with high negative stress or higher probability of injuries. It all depends on how fit a person is at that moment. A weightlifter isn't necessarily highly stressed when he lifts heavy weights because his muscles became strong enough after years of consistent training. However, if he's had an injury and hasn't trained for several weeks, his fitness level has dropped drastically, and even lighter weights could stress his sensitized structures. If he then progresses his training too quickly, the structures might not be able to catch up and might become irritated again.

Yet every activity can be tweaked in a way that won't overload our systems. Tweaking can be done by adjusting force, impact, duration, speed, or volume. This means that even though sitting doesn't seem like a high load for the body at first, sitting for eight hours a day can make it an extreme load for the body, causing lots of strain.

So if you've noticed that an activity is overloading your system because your body structures are irritated and you feel more tension or pain afterward, then consider tweaking the activity by shortening the duration, decreasing the speed, lowering the force or impact, or taking longer breaks in between.

When it comes to pain after exercising, it's very important to differentiate between *DOMS (delayed onset muscle soreness)* pain and sharp, uncomfortable pain. DOMS is the normal soreness we get after doing any activity our body hasn't done before or hasn't done at that intensity. That pain is totally acceptable whereas the sharp pain in the same area you usually have the pain (e.g., lower back) is feedback that some tweaking might be necessary.

If you repeatedly feel pain after your activities, some ways to specifically lower the load you put on your body are: doing challenging bodyweight instead of weight-lifting exercises; skipping those positions in your yoga class that excessively extend your spine; limiting time spent seated; or going for a run in the woods instead of on hard pavement.

On the other hand, we also know that a certain amount of load is necessary to build up our structures. Not exposing our bodies to the impact of walking or running will not build up strong, long lasting bones and fascia and might not get you doing your favorite activities again. Where can you tweak your activities to increase the load if you feel like your body isn't getting enough but actually is ready to take on some more?

PLANNING ACTIVITY PROGRESSION

Planning out our activities and progressions can save us from going through a lot of trial and error. Knowing and accepting our current fitness level and finding the sweet spot at which to load our system are the building blocks for that.

Thinking about reasonable progressions enables us to improve efficiently and safely at the same time. If you manage to progress gradually, you might be surprised at how well you feel after exposing your body to higher impact activities and how well the structures in the body, including bones and cartilage, can regenerate when you challenge them optimally.

However, when I started playing soccer again after eight years of never playing, even I didn't return so gradually at first. I sometimes played on very joint-straining surfaces for an hour without a break at a high intensity as if there were no tomorrow. And yet there was. While I felt only a little pain while playing, the next day it came up much stronger and stayed for one to two weeks. I kept thinking to myself: "Something must have broken again, and maybe I shouldn't play at all anymore." But no, the body just wasn't ready for that much load after not having played for such a long time.

When I planned my approach better and slowly increased the intensity, I was able to play a complete 90-minute soccer game again without pain, and, wonderfully, there was no pain in the days that followed. After more than eight years without this sport, it was very fulfilling for me to be able to kick the ball again without pain. That feeling alone helped me to empty my barrel sufficiently so that I know longer felt any pain.

So, when picking an activity that you want to optimize, think about what a reasonable progression would be and try to hold yourself back when you are exceeding that progression again.

Don't forget your recovery time. The body needs a certain amount of time to build up its structures again in order to make them as strong as before. If you do your next activity too early, those restorative measures aren't finished, and it can lead to overworking the body. While that recovery time is highly individual and depends on the fitness level of the person, using massages, sauna visits, meditation, relaxation techniques, or ice baths can speed up the recovery. So also take the time to give your body a nice treat after exposing it to high loads.

Action Steps:

1. **Determine what type you are.**

→ Be honest with yourself as you determine your current fitness level. Think about whether you usually overload your system, or whether you don't stimulate it enough to keep your body structures strong.

2. **Tweak your activities accordingly.**

→ Use the load variables to either decrease or increase the load you put on your system.

3. **Plan your activity progression.**

→ Pick an activity and think about a rational progression and adequate recovery time. Stick with the plan and don't let your emotions upset that plan.

MY APPRAISAL

The action steps of this area are especially appropriate for you if you tend to exaggerate when doing activities and if you often have more pain after certain activities. Also, if you usually don't think about how you can load your structures enough for them to stay strong in the long run or if you fear any type of load. If you have never made a plan that has also included recovery time in between the activity but rather would "wing it" when it came to sports and activities, this approach might be an opportunity for you to experience the benefits of preparation and planning. In these cases, select a higher number for the first question about your conviction.

How convinced are you that the action steps in this area can help you?
On a scale of 1-10:

0	1	2	3	4	5	6	7	8	9	10

How inspired are you to do the action steps?
On a scale of 1-10:

0	1	2	3	4	5	6	7	8	9	10

How likely you are you to implement the action steps?
On a scale of 1-10:

0	1	2	3	4	5	6	7	8	9	10

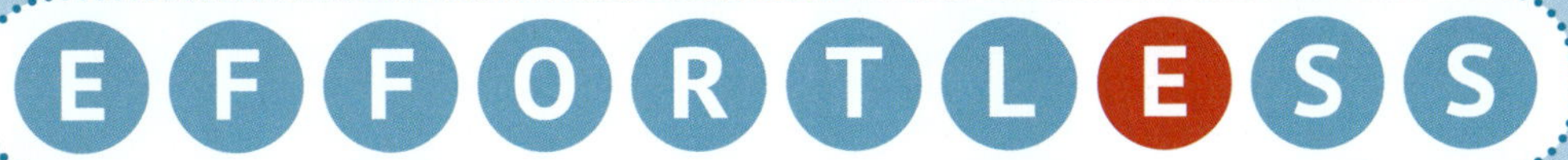

3.3.8 ERGONOMICS

When it comes to ergonomics at the workplace, there are several things to consider, from the light, noises, and radiation we're exposed to, to the posture we're in, the shoes we wear, and the loads we must lift. As far as improving our back health is concerned, our main goal is to facilitate an optimal posture in which we have the least wear and tear or compression on the spine. I've always thought that ergonomics was just for the elderly and I didn't need to pay attention to it because I was young and fit. Despite the back problems I suffered for years, I would never really consider changing anything about the way I sat throughout the day. I thought I just had bad luck with my back, and, apart from a few exercises, I couldn't do anything about it anyway.

But after years spending a lot of time on my laptop in libraries, I realized just how not ergonomic our student environment was. The tables were too low, the laptops weren't used with any elevation, and the chairs made sitting in a balanced position impossible. No wonder more and more students are complaining about back pain and neck tensions. Even when you're at a younger age, you don't have an oversized barrel in which hours of poor ergonomic work and exam stress fits in easily.

Students often sit in a library for much longer than a normal workload for an office worker, and nobody there cares about ergonomics. That's why I got creative and decided to create as best as I could an almost proper ergonomic workplace using the basket. (see fig. 3.74). So if we don't get the best ergonomic workstation from our employer, instead of only complaining about it, we can get creative and put certain objects on the table or floor, find a wall that we lean against, or use specific equipment like a laptop stand to follow good ergonomic standards.

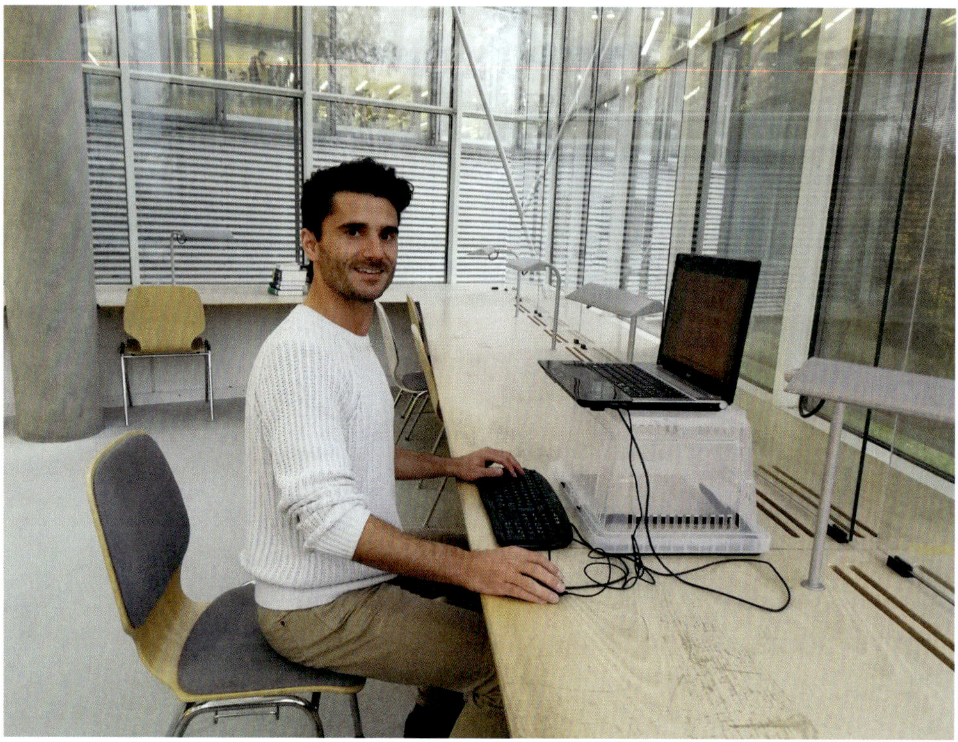

Fig. 3.74: My self-built ergonomic workstation in the library

Because of the load on our bodies that comes from sitting for 7 or 8 hours at a desk every day, ergonomic interventions can make a big difference. Those interventions aim to reduce biomechanical strain caused by ergonomic or organizational changes at work and in the working environment. A person should always follow ergonomic standards when sitting at a desk (fig. 3.75).

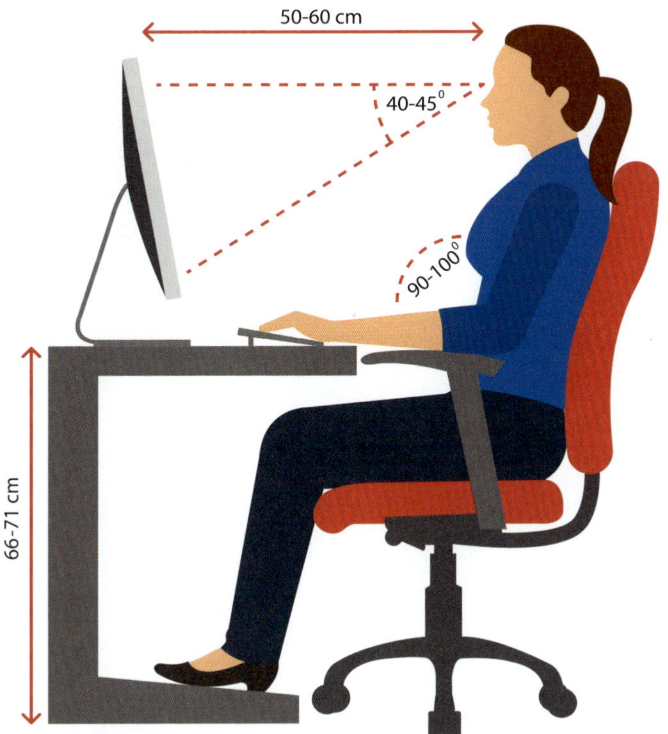

Fig. 3.75: Ergonomic seat

- table height between about 26-28 inches (66-71 cm)
- the eyes are at the height of the upper edge of the screen
- distance to the screen is 20-24 inches (50-60 cm)
- elbow joint should be at 90 to 100 degrees
- right angle in the knee joint or the knees point slightly downward
- Be sure that the screen is not too reflective and is at least 19 inches in size, so that the room is bright enough and evenly lit, and that the backrest, seat height, and armrests of the chair are adjustable.

Fortunately, nowadays more and more employees own a height-adjustable worktable. Ideally, on a regular office day, the standing desk should be used 30% of the time, whereas sitting should still make up 60% and moving 10%. Although the change between sitting and standing is already very healthy for our back, ergonomics should also be considered with the standing desk (fig. 3.76).

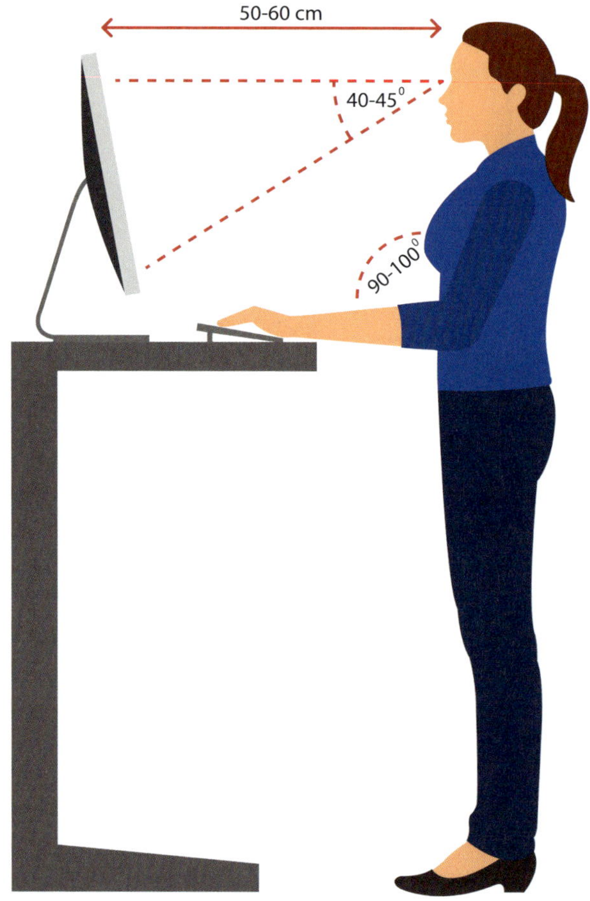

Fig. 3.76: Standing desk

- Stand in front of the desk and let the forearms rest on the table surface.
- Your shoulders are relaxed, not raised toward the ears.
- Your feet are standing firmly on the floor and weight is evenly distributed. One foot can occasionally be placed on a footrest.
- The bend at the elbows is approximately 90 degrees.
- The screen is raised so that your eyes are at the same level as the top of the screen.

For movement and transfer tasks at the workplace, the circumstances can also be made more ergonomic (see fig. 3.77).

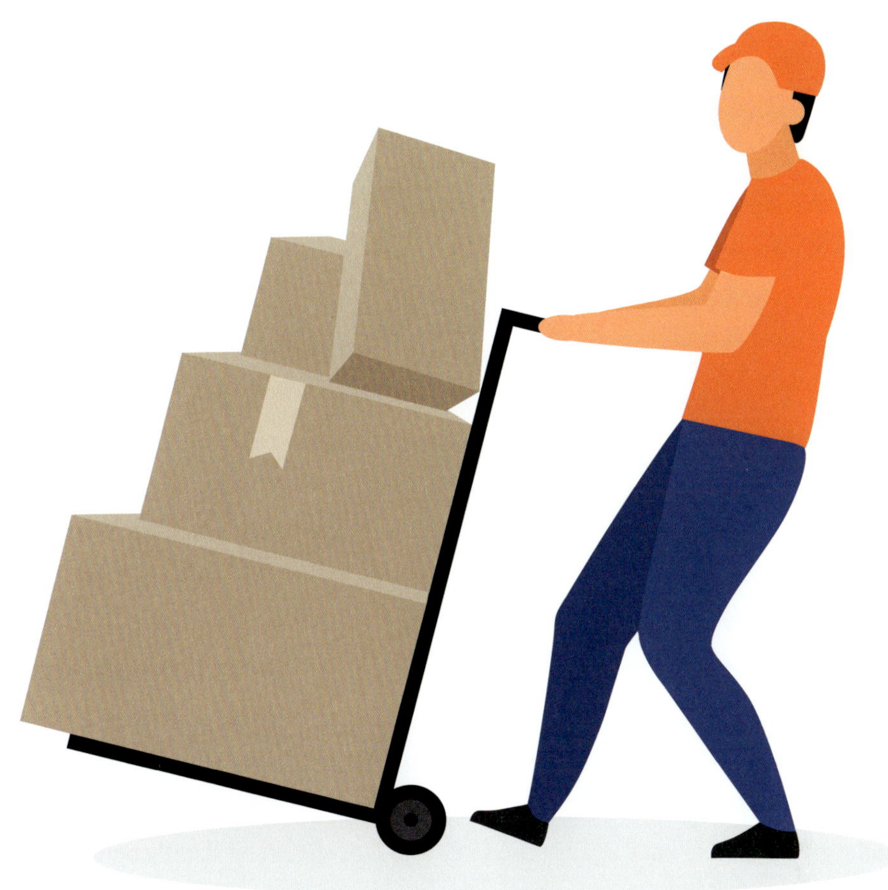

Fig. 3.77: Ergonomics during movement and transfer tasks

- Use simple aids such as sack trucks, slings, roller boards, glide mats, belts, roller systems, and lifting aids.
- Lift trucks or forklifts make manual lifting and carrying loads unnecessary.
- The use of technical lifting and carrying aids, such as pallet truck manipulators, lifts, and cranes, are further options.
- Reduce vibrations and shocks in vehicles (e.g., forklift trucks).

For many people, driving a car is also a daily activity. These people often suffer from back problems due to a lack of ergonomics, too. Pain can be avoided by correctly adjusting the seat and using some additional tricks (see fig. 3.78).

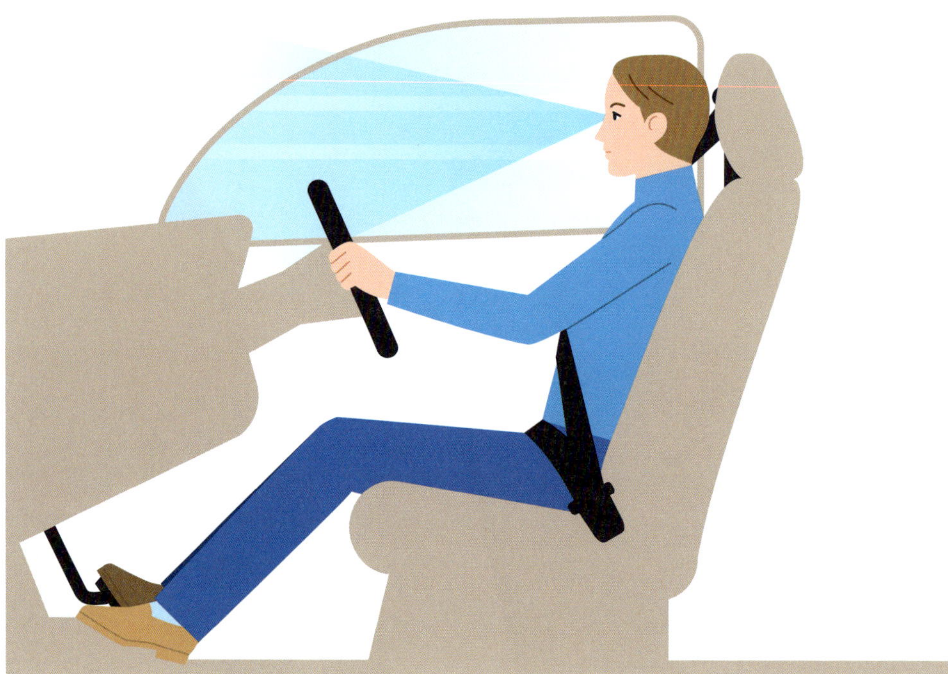

Fig. 3.78: Driving seat

- Adjust the backrest so that the steering wheel can be reached with the arms slightly bent, and the shoulders can maintain contact with the seat even when steering.
- Sit with your entire back against the seat. Your legs should be slightly bent when the gas pedal is pressed.
- Adjust the seat height so that there is a handbreadth of space between your head and the headrest.
- Adjust the seat height so that your thighs rest loosely and point straight forward or slightly down, while your butt remains in contact with the back.
- The length of the seat should be adjusted so that there is a space of two to three finger widths between the back of your knees and the front edge of the seat.
- Your pelvis should be slightly tilted as in the "balanced sitting position." A small lumbar support could help you here.
- The side guides of the seat should support the upper body at the sides, but should not press against it.
- Adjust the headrest so that the head is protected but the neck is not. The upper edge of the headrest should be at the same level as the upper edge of the head.

LEARNING BALANCED POSTURES

I observed, though, that when people tried to sit upright at their desks, they usually had at least one thing they hadn't thought of that kept them from following those optimal ergonomic standards. Maybe the text on the screen was too small and they couldn't really see it well enough, so they moved their heads forward slightly, or they weren't able to freely write without having to look down at the keyboard all the time, overstraining the neck, or their jeans were so tight that they couldn't breathe into their lower belly. But those small changes that altered an ideal sitting position can change the tensions in the whole body, leading to overloading certain parts.

So, in order to get into the "optimal" posture, besides having an ergonomic workplace, it also helps to know exactly how that posture feels. When we're really sitting in a balanced sitting position, we feel as if we can remain in it easily. If we are tense in any part of the body, the position may look "straight," but it's not the balanced sitting position. On the other hand, if you don't feel like you can be perfectly straight but it still feels effortless to sit this way, then this probably is your balanced sitting posture. Often our own perception of what feels straight doesn't really look straight and vice versa. If you use a mirror or ask someone to tell you what looks straight, you might be surprised. To get into a balanced sitting posture on a chair, follow the instructions in fig. 3.79.

Note: In order to assume the balanced sitting position, it is helpful to carry out the individual training program from section 3.4 beforehand, as this aims to create a balance in the tension between the front and rear muscle chains, which simplifies the balanced sitting position.

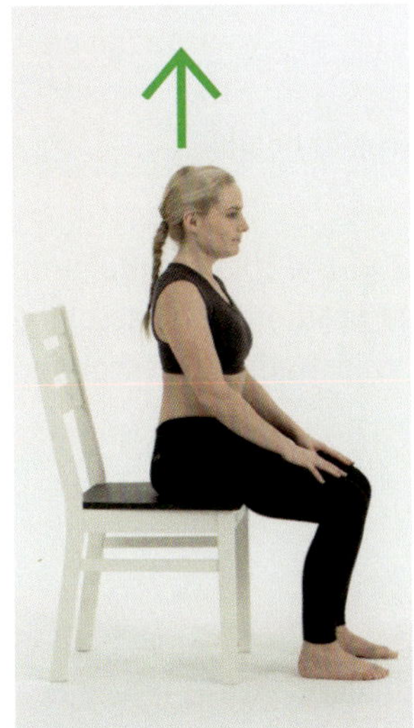

Fig. 3.79: Balanced sitting on chair

Stand in front of a chair, tilt the pelvis, push the butt back, and then sit on the front half of the chair. The chair should be at such a height that the knees are at a 90-degree angle or point down slightly. Feet and knees point straight forward, and the pelvis should be slightly tilted so that you feel the front edge of your sit bones. The rib cage is positioned directly above the pelvis, and the shoulders are opened wide, which keeps them from lifting into the ears. Lower your chin until about the length of a fist can fit between your chin and sternum, stretching your neck as if someone were pulling you long by the back of your head. Then, try to consciously relax your back, abdominal, and neck muscles without changing position. In this sitting position, breathe consciously into your abdomen and lower rib cage so that they expand in all directions as you inhale.

The strategies for healthier sitting can also be transferred to other postures in everyday life, such as standing, sleeping, lifting, or a slight hip hinge like, for example, when vacuuming. Standing for long periods of time in the same position can lead to tension, as can lying in an unfavorable position or vacuuming with a rounded back.

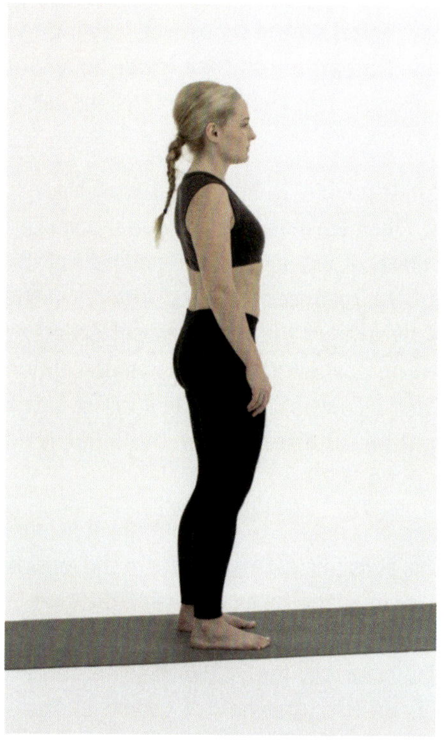

Fig. 3.80: Balanced standing posture

Stand upright in a hip-width position. Point your toes forward and bend your knees slightly. Try to distribute the pressure evenly over your heels and the outside and inside of the balls of your feet. Tilt your pelvis forward slightly so that it sits right above the ankles and the rib cage is positioned directly above the pelvis. The shoulders are opened wide, which keeps them from lifting into the ears. Lower your chin until about the length of a fist can fit between your chin and sternum, while stretching your neck as if someone was pulling you long by the back of your head. Then, try to consciously relax your back, abdominal, and neck muscles without changing position. In this standing position, breathe consciously into your abdomen and lower rib cage so that they expand in all directions as you inhale.

In the sleeping positions (see figs. 3.81, 3.82, and 3.83), none of the three is preferred over the other because the cues in those allow the neutral sine position to be assumed in each. So, stick with your favorite sleeping position and try to just adjust it according to the images.

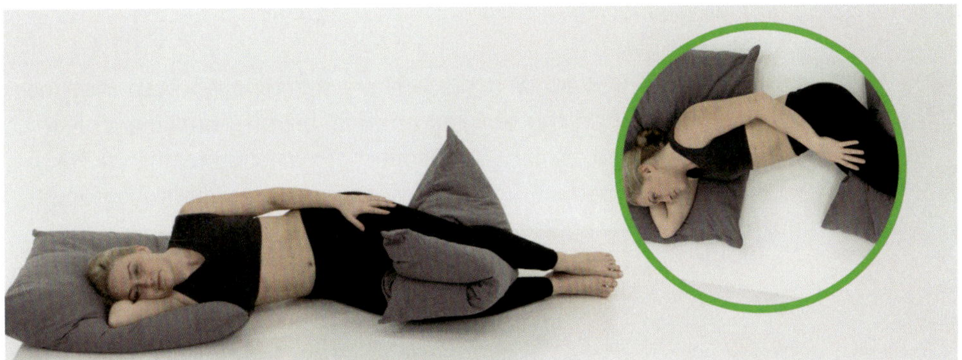

Fig. 3.81: Lateral sleeping position

Lie down on your side and position your head on a pillow that is high enough so your head rests at the same level as the spine. You can position your bent or stretched arm under the pillow or head and place your upper arm on your pelvis or in front of you. The upper shoulder will be held low so that it is as far away from your ear as possible. Your head lies stretched out on the pillow so that about the length of a fist can fit between your chin and sternum. Keep your entire back in its neutral position while tilting your pelvis forward slightly and flexing your knees and pelvis to about 120 degrees. If necessary, place a second cushion between your knees to protect them. In this sleeping position, breathe into your stomach and lower rib cage so that they expand in all directions when you breathe in. Try to consciously relax your entire body.

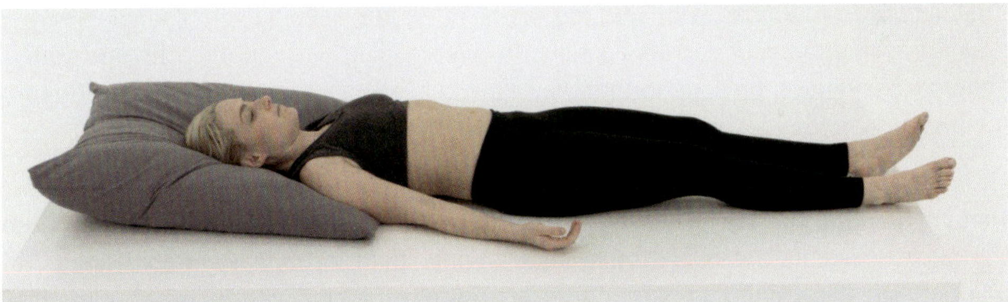

Fig. 3.82: Supine sleeping position

Lie on your back and position your head and shoulders on a pillow that is high enough for your head to rest at the same level as the spine. Your head lies stretched out on the pillow so that about the length of a fist can fit between your chin and sternum. Keep the shoulders low so that they are as far away from the ears as possible. The arms rest next to your body while the hands are turned up as much as possible.

(continued)

Supine sleeping position (continued)

The pelvis is slightly tilted forward, and the legs are slightly opened so that the feet are turned outward a bit. In this sleeping position, breathe into your stomach and lower rib cage so that they expand in all directions as you breathe in. Try to consciously relax your entire body. If you still feel increased tension in your lower back, you can also put a pillow under the backs of your knees.

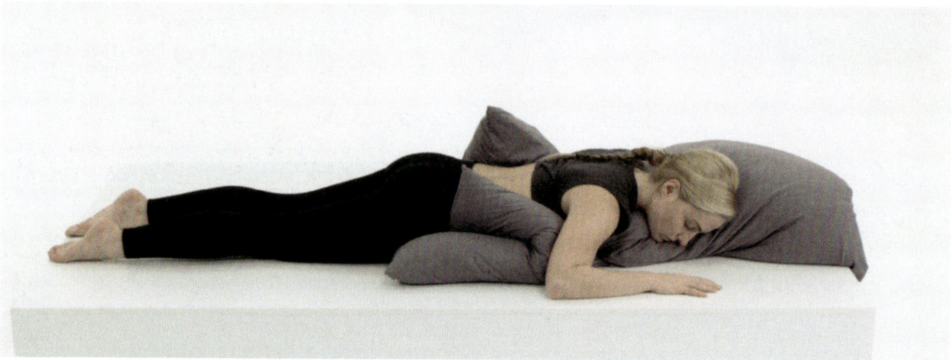

Fig. 3.83: Prone sleeping position

Lie facedown in the prone position. Place a pillow under your stomach if you feel too much tension in your lower back. Place one side of your face on the pillow so that it points diagonally downward and the neck is not turned too much. Put your hands above your head with your elbows pointing out, keeping your shoulders low, as far away from your ears as possible. In this sleeping position, breathe into your stomach and lower rib cage so that they expand in all directions as you inhale. Try to consciously relax your entire body.

Hinging from the hip (see fig. 3.84) is more efficient than bending from the back because the large hip joints are more stable and stronger than individual vertebral joints. In addition, the hamstring and gluteal muscles can also be activated by pushing the hips back, where the loads are better distributed over the entire myofascial back line. If we adopt such a position while, for example, vacuuming or wiping the floor over a long period of time, then it makes sense to always choose the hip hinge as the starting position.

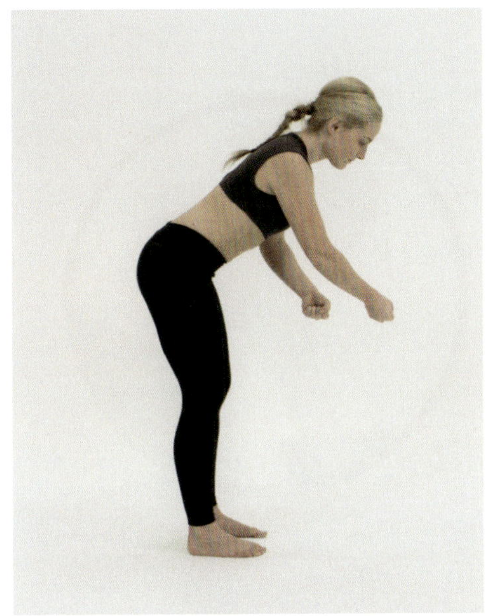

Fig. 3.84: Hinging from the hip

Stand with feet shoulder-width apart and knees slightly bent. Then, tilt your pelvis forward slightly, push your butt back, and lean your upper body forward slightly while keeping your spine in its neutral position. From this position, any work, such as sweeping the floor or shoveling, can be carried out in a more back-friendly way.

Usually we're taught to pick up heavy objects with a straight spine and bent knees. Even though this method can also put a lot of stress on the knees if optimal technique is missing, it is generally the most efficient, spine-sparing way to lift (see fig. 3.85).

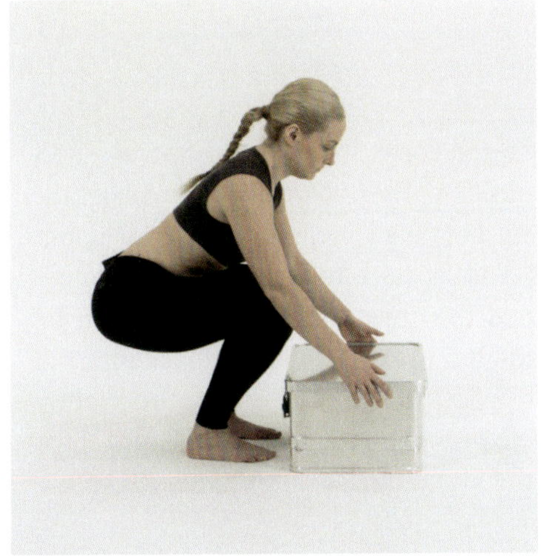

Fig. 3.85: Picking up a heavy object

Stand directly in front of the heavy object. Feet and knees should point forward, and the entire spine should be in its neutral position. Distribute the weight evenly between your heels and the outside and inside of the balls of your feet. Then, tilt your pelvis forward slightly, push your butt back, and slowly lower your body as far as you can while still holding your entire spine in its natural position. Then grasp the object with both hands, tense your gluteal and abdominal muscles, and push yourself up using your legs.

Since injuries in the back often occur when the spine is in a twisted position, it is wise to also learn a more spine-sparing technique, especially when picking up heavy things (see fig. 3.86).

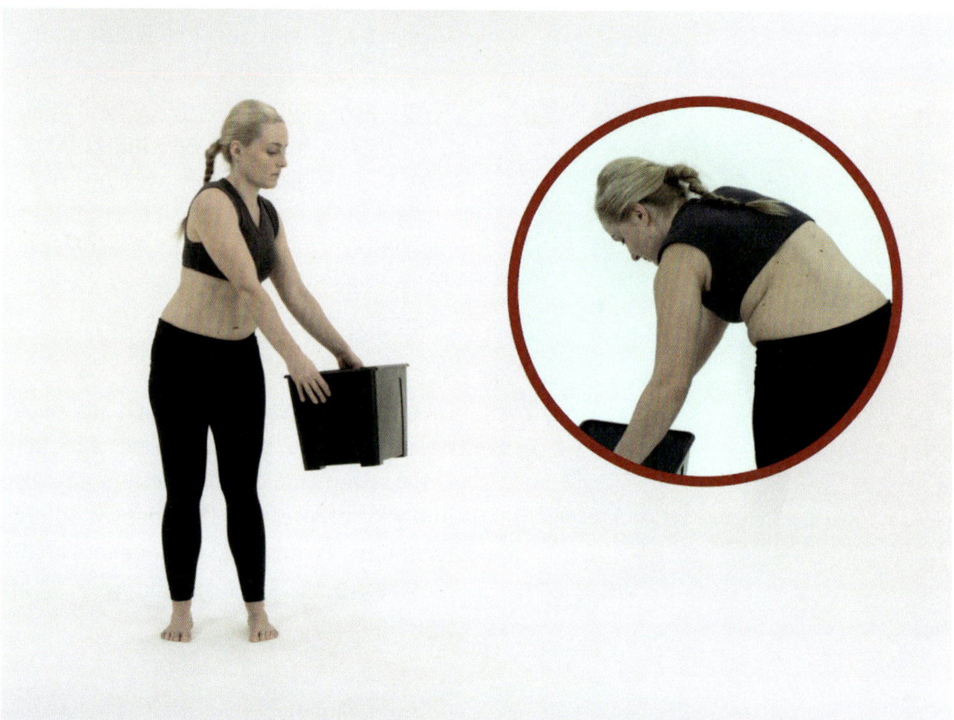

Fig. 3.86: Picking up an object with a rotary motion

Stand directly in front of the object. Your feet and knees should point forward, and your entire spine should be in its neutral position. Then, bend your legs slightly, tilt your pelvis forward slightly, and push your butt back while hinging your upper body forward. If necessary, bend the knees a little more to keep the entire spine in its neutral position. Once you have grasped the object, straighten up again by pushing your hips forward. Then turn from the hip to the side to get back into the starting position. To put the object back on the floor, tilt your pelvis forward slightly again, push your butt back, and lower while your upper body remains forward. Take particular care not to turn your back during the lifting movement (see red circle).

DYNAMIC SITTING AND FREE MOVEMENTS

Even though balanced sitting can, if done correctly, decrease the strain on the body, resting in any posture for too long can still lead to problems. By focusing on dynamic sitting, we make sure that certain muscles aren't overloaded by remaining stationary for too long and that the blood can circulate through the body.

If circumstances prevent us from sitting in a balanced position because maybe the chair is just too low, the screen too high, or the sofa too soft, and there's nothing to tweak to get to the optimal ergonomic standard, then it´s pointless and sometimes even counterproductive to strive for the balanced sitting position in the first place as this can lead to increased tension. In that case, skip even trying to get into a balanced sitting position but instead go for dynamic sitting and only focus on changing your sitting position as often as possible (at least every 20 minutes).

You might also notice that some sitting positions relieve your pain whereas others trigger them. Since everyone's bodies are different, play around with different postures and use those postures which relieve pain.

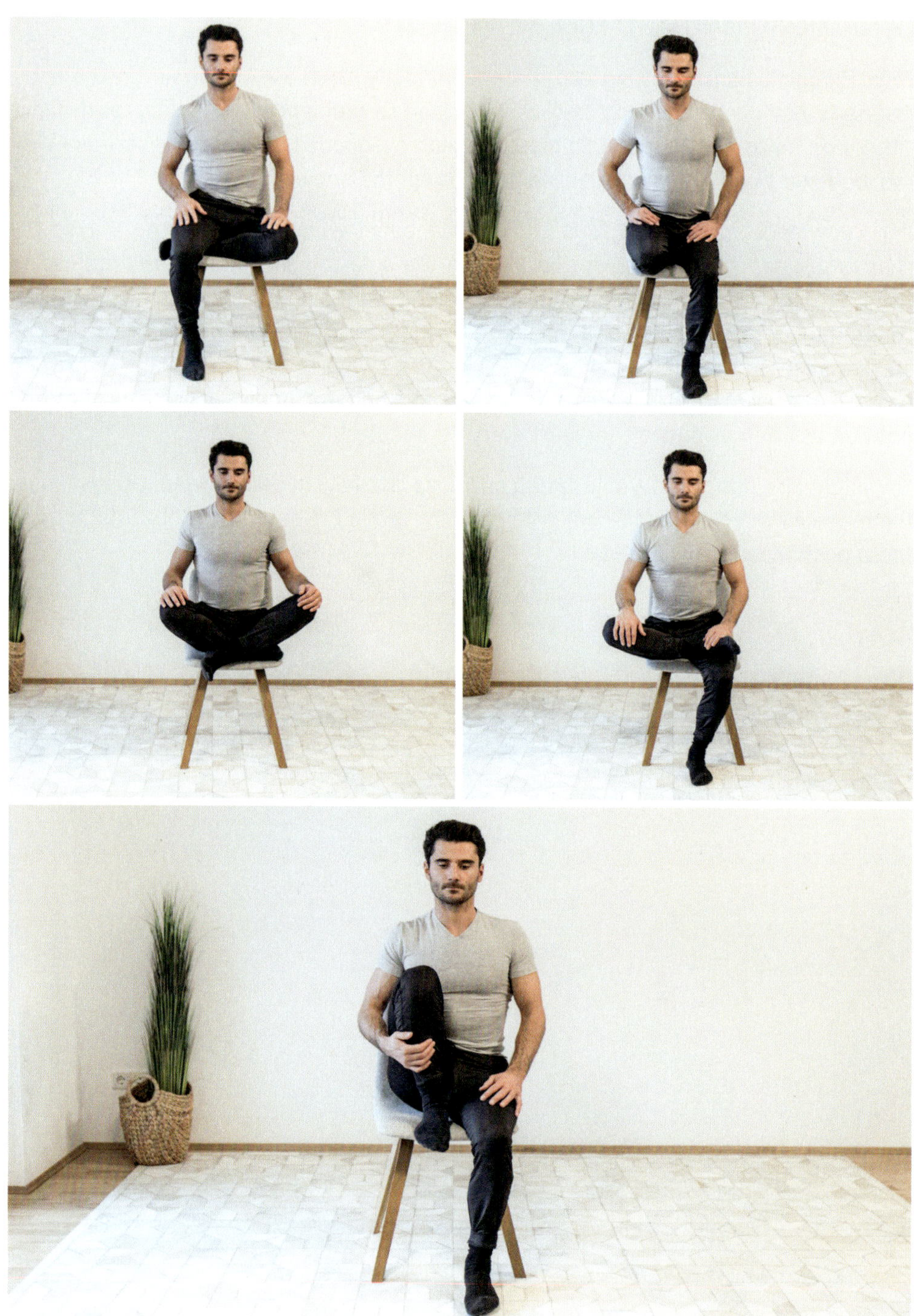

Fig. 3.87: Different leg positions in dynamic sitting

During dynamic sitting, the sitting posture is changed so frequently that the muscles do not even begin to tense. So when we sit dynamically, we move from one sitting position to the next, true to the motto: The next sitting posture is the best sitting posture. The backrest, the side supports, or the table can always be used to lean on to decrease the compression on the back, but also changing positions of the legs as in these examples is worthwhile, as the motion moves fluid through the legs while preserving hip flexibility at the same time.

The same also applies to standing as well as the sleeping position. Try to take the balanced position as a starting point and move out of it in a variety of ways. As far as sleeping is concerned, we move out of the initial position at some point during the night anyway, but falling asleep in a comfortable position is key here.

In order to get feedback about your posture, you can also use posture sensor devices on your clothes that remind you to adjust your posture and move more. There are even chairs now that check if you move enough and remind you whenever you don't.

Hinges, squats, or other movements in everyday life usually only become a problem if they're accompanied by an individual compensatory pattern (see section 2.2.2). For example, a construction worker always works with the same technique and compensates for his lack of hip mobility by predominantly moving a certain area in his back. In those cases, it might be important to learn to use more ergonomic techniques as shown previously. But other than that, it's wise to concentrate on moving as freely as you can, trying out many movement variations.

The key here is to find the sweet spot where you challenge the muscles and the fascia of your back, but don't overload them with either repeated, one-sided movements or new heavy loads.

MY APPRAISAL

The activities of this area are especially appropriate for you if you lack ergonomics and movement in your everyday life, if you often wake up in the morning with tension or pain, if you don't sleep well in general, or if you notice that your approach to persevere in an upright posture often leads to even more tension. In these cases, select a higher number for the first question about your conviction.

Action steps:

1. **Improve ergonomics in one chosen area.**

→ Think of where you would need better ergonomics in your everyday life: at work, while driving, or at home? Pick one are and implement suitable ergonomics.

2. **Practice the balanced postures you need.**

→ Think about in which everyday positions learning balanced postures is necessary. Practice the ergonomic postures until you have internalized them.

3. **Focus on moving more.**

→ Use dynamic sitting and standing whenever the balanced option is not possible or has been used for too long. Also set a reminder to move more in general.

How convinced are you that the action steps in this area can help you? On a scale of 1-10:

0	1	2	3	4	5	6	7	8	9	10

How inspired are you to do the action steps? On a scale of 1-10:

0	1	2	3	4	5	6	7	8	9	10

How likely are you to implement the action steps? On a scale of 1-10:

0	1	2	3	4	5	6	7	8	9	10

E F F O R T L E S S

3.3.9 STRESS MANAGEMENT

Minimizing negative stress is the key ability in our modern, stressful lives. If we learn how to do that, and bring balance back into our minds, we empty the bedrock of our barrel. In order to minimize the influence of stressors respectively to learn to cope with negative stress, there are three different method levels:

1. The instrumental level.

The aim is to reduce stress factors by changing the external stresses and demands. Better time management, delegation, or structuring are intended to eliminate time pressure, communication, problems and overstrain in professional and family life.

2. The cognitive level.

This includes the previously described cognitive restructuring to change our motivation as well as to change patterns of thinking, attitude, and perception.

3. The palliative-regenerative level.

This is about relieving physical and psychological stress symptoms. For small, everyday activities, such as walking, meeting friends, or other leisure activities, targeted relaxation and stress reduction methods, such as progressive muscle relaxation, autogenic training, or meditation, can be used.

While the palliative–regenerative level probably includes the simplest and most comfortable methods, the other two involve a little more effort. However, the causes of stress are more likely to be tackled at these levels, which is why more sustainable effects can be expected here. On the cognitive level, there's even the possibility of transforming distress into eustress, which is the best way to empty the barrel.

While acute, major stress factors, such as the loss of a job, a death in the family, or the separation of a partner, can be easily identified, it is the latent, subliminal stress factors that are often not properly perceived as such by us. While during acute stress the relationship to the physical complaints can be quickly established, latent stress gradually fills our barrel in the long run. This can also include worries, fears of loss, or unfulfilled wishes.

A targeted analysis of the stress factors is important in order to identify both the acute, conscious stress factors and the hidden, latent ones.

To determine your latent stress, write down what your biggest stress factors are. Think about you and your life. What exactly is stressing you? It could be, for example, the relationship with a colleague at work, a friend, or a partner; the flood of tasks at work; an exam situation in which you "have to" present yourself; a situation in the future about you constantly worry about; problems with technology; or decisions which you are unsure about.

METHODS TO MANAGE STRESS

In order to get rid of your biggest stress factor, you first need to prioritize the stressors. Which stress factor is most meaningful to you? Which one has the greatest influence on filling your barrel? Which one do you want to get rid of fast?

Starting with the stress factor number one helps the most because when the biggest stress factor has already been resolved, the biggest part of the barrel is emptied, and the world already looks completely different. Once you've decided on the most important stress factor, here is how you can resolve the stress on each of the three levels:

1. Instrumental method.

Think about which problems can be solved by rejecting them. To do this, you will think of a strategy that you can use to delegate work tasks, optimize your schedule, reject requests, allow yourself more time, or clarify something important in a conversation. Write the options next to it and decide on one.

You can even meditate on possible solutions. Ask yourself: "How can I get rid of that stressor?" Maybe you have to push yourself to be able to say no to people. You might be surprised, though, that the consequences of that are sometimes not as bad as we expect them to be.

2. Cognitive method.

Try to change your attitude and perception toward the stress factor because, as we have learned, people react to stress factors in many ways. For example, if you're standing in a long line in a grocery store, you can either get irritated (even if you're not even in a hurry) and cause your blood pressure to increase, or just grab a magazine that you really wanted to flip through and be grateful for the time to read it without having to buy it. In most cases, we get into something without seeing or understanding the other side and discovering the possibilities in it.

With the following exercise you can go through your stress factors and neutralize them by doing some mental work. To do this, create a table (see table 3.1) and write your worst expectation regarding the stress situation in the first column.

Then list all the advantages that this fear would bring if it were to become reality in the second and third columns. In columns two and three, you then add the secondary and other additional advantages, those that would then arise from it. Search again for advantages in all seven areas of life.

These include:

1. the professional area
2. the financial area
3. the family area
4. the physical area
5. the social area
6. the mental area
7. the spiritual area

List as many advantages as possible and keep in mind that an advantage is also something we can learn from the situation. Of course, the benefits are all purely hypothetical, but so, too, are the drawbacks we fear.

Through this exercise, you can change your perception of the expected outcome so that you don't see the result as just negative and threatening, but also as something beneficial that presents new opportunities. So don't stop the exercise until you have noticed that the situation is no longer stressing you negatively.

Stress situation: Working at a desk for too long.

Tab. 3.1: Sample list for solving a stressful situation using the cognitive approach

Fears	Benefits	Secondary benefits	Additional benefits
I can't do all the work and lose the project.	I can learn to better prioritize or delegate.	I can do what suits me better.	I can live my full potential.
	I learn to only take on tasks that I can manage.	I'm learning to say no.	I don't live by other people's plans.
	I don't have to work overtime, and I have more free time.	My spouse is glad that I have more time again.	I can save my marriage that way.
	I'm learning to get by with less money.	I'm cutting unnecessary expenses.	I'm gaining more control over my finances.
	I don't have to deal with annoying customers anymore.	I no longer take the conflicts home with me and will sleep better.	I can empty my barrel, and my back becomes healthier.

In this example, one could think that finding all the benefits of not being able to do all the work would prevent us from continuing to work meticulously. Quite the opposite is the case, actually, because it wouldn't necessarily defeat our goal of "getting stuff done," but rather doing this exercise helps us to work more efficiently and with more focus because we don't always have our worst fear in mind, which stresses us and fills our barrel.

After you've found sufficient advantages for the first worry, repeat the process with your next worry until you realize that the whole situation no longer stresses you negatively.

3. Palliative–regenerative method.

With this approach, think about how you could treat yourself regularly to recover from the stressful situations and (at least temporarily) empty your barrel. This could be possible through conversations, coping through physical activity, distraction by doing hobbies or using media entertainment options, as well as relaxation methods such as progressive muscle relaxation, sauna, or meditation.

ELIMINATING THE BIGGEST STRESS FACTOR

Thinking about which method to pick is very important in order to increase the chances of its success. Here are some things to consider when picking the right method.

Using method number 1 could be the fastest way to resolve the stressor, so this approach is worthwhile. However, it can sometimes be hard to overcome inner blocks in order to say no to people, to delegate tasks, or to allow more time for certain projects. If you're ready for that challenge, this might be your best approach.

Method number 2 needs a lot of mental work and challenges your sometimes deep-rooted perceptions of things. But once you've understood the concept and it starts to work, you will have a method that you can use for the rest of your life. So it will definitely be worth it to put in the time and mental work.

For some people, taking out the time to take care for their own recovery is a big challenge as well because they usually don't give themselves permission to do so and instead keep on pushing themselves to stay active. For those people, especially, method number 3 can be the best option, but the other two methods address the causes of the stressors and are more likely to empty the barrel sustainably.

MY APPRAISAL

This area is especially appropriate for you if you have noticed that your back problems occur mainly when you are stressed an if you feel that your barrel is generally quite full and you must cope with great burden. In these cases, select a higher number for the first question about your conviction.

Action steps:

1. **Analyze stress factors.**

→ List all the stress factors you currently have in your life, the obvious ones as well as the hidden, underlying one.

2. **Prioritize the stress factors.**

→ Prioritize your list of stress factors according to how great their influence is on you.

3. **Choose a method and resolve the stress.**

→ Pick the biggest stress factor and choose a method to resolve it.

How convinced are you that the action steps in this area can help you?
On a scale of 1-10:

0	1	2	3	4	5	6	7	8	9	10

How inspired are you to do the action steps?
On a scale of 1-10:

0	1	2	3	4	5	6	7	8	9	10

How likely are you to implement the action steps?
On a scale of 1-10:

0	1	2	3	4	5	6	7	8	9	10

E F F O R T L E S **S**

3.3.10 SOCIAL SUPPORT

As we learned in the chapter 2, having supportive, caring, but not overly concerned people around us can really help us to empty the barrel. Although this book is about independence and self-empowerment, it makes sense to not close ourselves completely to the help of others. Just as the passive methods described in the section 3.6 can support us on our way to sustained back health, so, too, can the support of social contacts.

If there's someone, though, who is all about doom and gloom, telling you the things you should worry about, you could consider either telling them to stop because you know this could facilitate your nocebo effect, or you could try not spending that much time with them. Instead surround yourself with people who are more positive, perhaps who also have success stories about how they overcame their own back pain. Hearing about their successes will help you trust in your ability to succeed.

When considering the great effect social interactions have on our health, we should consider setting goals for our social interactions just as we set training goals. When we reach those goals and have fulfilling social interactions, that fulfillment will certainly empty the barrel. Meeting up with friends twice a week, attending some inspiring events, or going out again can be goals we set. Before we can set those goals, though, we need to know what exact result we want. Is it more social interaction in general but eliminating the nocebo-inducing influence of others, or contacts who support our attempts to change certain aspects of our lives?

SOCIAL SUPPORT FOR ACHIEVEMENTS

Motivational speakers often say, "you're the average of the five people you spend the most time with." Our friends, then, might have a bigger influence on our behavior than we sometimes want to admit. Why? Because our mirror neurons in our brain make us subconsciously copy their behavior. When we plan to eat a healthy diet and everyone at work is eating unhealthily, we have to assert even more effort to go against what our mirror neurons tell us to do. So, in order to achieve a goal for a behavior change, it is helpful to surround ourselves with like-minded people or at least communicate to the people we can't exclude from our everyday life that we would like them to appreciate and respect our new behavior (e.g., we don't want them to offer us sweets at work all the time). Maybe there is even someone who could actively support us by teaming up with us and pursuing a healthy diet together, someone who can give us tips or tell us about their experiences, or someone who prepares healthy lunches for himself every day and would be happy to share it with us.

If we take on a goal that strongly challenges us, encouragement and energetic support from our social circle can inspire us. If we don't get that support, though, we might end up using it as an excuse for why we couldn't achieve our goals.

But oftentimes, we are too proud, shy, or stubborn to ask our colleagues, partners, or friends for support, even though they might be very happy to support us and would feel fulfilled if they could help.

SUPPORTING OTHERS HELPS OUR HEALTH AS WELL

If we don't have enough social support, it could be because we are not reciprocating and showing others support and encouragement. Maybe we haven't called our friends in a long time and asked them what we could do for them. By focusing on doing those things again, we can increase our chances to engage in social interactions once more.

Giving others support will help us empty our barrel because it increases positive feelings, activates the reward centers in the brain, and deactivates the threat centers. It is a win-win situation to care for others as well ourselves. So try texting or calling that neglected friend and simply ask how he or she is doing. Or even create a little get-together and invite all your old friends.

Also, if we want to ask a person for support on our way to achieving a goal, it can be helpful if we consider beforehand how we can help that person in ways that are important to them, making it easier to ask for something in return. If there is something you want to do with them together, show them what's in it for them. That will open them up to support you in that endeavor.

MY APPRAISAL

This area is especially appropriate for you if you spend a lot of time with people who have a rather unhealthy lifestyle, tell you only about the bad things happening to them, or if you don't have many social contacts in general and feel socially isolated. Also, this area is good if you know you will need support to achieve a certain goal such as seeing the back-health plan of this book through. In these cases, select a higher number for the first question about your conviction.

Action steps:

1. **Determine what support you need.**

→ Think about what exactly you would need social support for with regard to your holistic back health.
Do you need more social interaction in general? More empowering connections? Or do you need specific support to achieve a certain goal? Who will be those people?

2. **Think of what's in it for them.**

→ Then think about how you can do something for them in order to ask for something in return.

3. **Create a plan for how to approach them.**

→ Think beforehand how you will approach the person and try to communicate your request by showing them how they will benefit from it as well.

How convinced are you that the action steps in this area can help you?
On a scale of 1-10:

0	1	2	3	4	5	6	7	8	9	10

How inspired are you to do the action steps?
On a scale of 1-10:

0	1	2	3	4	5	6	7	8	9	10

How likely are you to implement the action steps?
On a scale of 1-10:

0	1	2	3	4	5	6	7	8	9	10

4 YOUR INDIVIDUAL BACK-HEALTH PLAN

Now that you have become familiar with all the action steps within the different areas, it's time to create your individual back-health plan. The simple act of creating a plan and visualizing the integration of the action steps into your everyday life activates your "executive center" (Prefrontal Cortex) in your brain which is responsible for bringing order and organization into your life and suppressing your distracting impulses and your "weaker self." So take the time to think about your answers in each of the 10 areas again while you fill in the following sections to determine your plan.

Transfer the EFFORTLESS scores from each of the 10 areas and create a ranking, starting with number one for the highest score.

Tab. 4.1: Create your back health plan

Your back-health plan

EFFORTLESS area	EFFORTLESS score	Rank
Exercises Action Step 1: Do the self-tests and choose the exercises accordingly.		
Action Step 2: Try the exercises out.		
Action Step 3: Tweak the plan and train regularly.		
Favorite Activity Action Step 1: Find your favorite activity.		
Action Step 2: Prepare it.		

(continued)

(continued)

EFFORTLESS area	EFFORTLESS score	Rank
Action Step 3: Warm up and be brave enough to do it.		
Fuel Action Step 1: Pick one big thing and change it.		
Action Step 2: Exchange one inflammatory food with one anti-inflammatory food.		
Action Step 3: Change one behavior.		
Optimizing Environment Action Step 1: Include more NEAT activities at work.		
Action Step 2: Eliminate obstacles and excuses.		
Action Step 3: Emphasize better regeneration at home.		
Reason Determination Action Step 1: Find the reason behind your pain.		

EFFORTLESS area	EFFORTLESS score	Rank
Action Step 2: Find the reasons for your back health.		
Action Step 3: Visualize your reasons.		
Treatments Action Step 1: Search for suitable treatments.		
Action Step 2: Research each treatment and select one.		
Action Step 3: Ask for activity recommendations.		
Load Management Action Step 1: Determine what type you are.		
Action Step 2: Tweak your activities accordingly.		
Action Step 3: Plan your activity progression.		
Ergonomics Action Step 1: Improve ergonomics in one chosen area.		

(continued)

(continued)

EFFORTLESS area	EFFORTLESS score	Rank
Action Step 2: Practice the balanced postures you need.		
Action Step 3: Focus on moving more.		
Stress Management Action Step 1: Analyze stress factors.		
Action Step 2: Prioritize the stress factors.		
Action Step 3: Choose a method and resolve the stress.		
Social Support Action Step 1: Determine what support you need.		
Action Step 2: Think of what's in it for them.		
Action Step 3: Create a plan for how to approach them.		

4.1 SETTING REALISTIC GOALS

When it comes to setting goals for our own health, most people do it superficially and don't really think it through which is why they fail on the way to implementation. For the method in this book to work, the tips and exercises must be implemented consistently. The EFFORTLESS method supports you in choosing the right action steps that suit you and your lifestyle best. But it's also important to set the right goals for implementing your back-health plan.

In general, you should try to carry out the action steps that are ranked 1 through 3, but as already described in section 3.1, you can also start with one or two areas first, if that would be more realistic for you so that you don't under- or overload yourself.

Oftentimes, we set unrealistic goals which we can't meet and blame ourselves until we eventually stop setting goals anymore at all. Without goals, though, we don't know how to move forward. To get out of that vicious circle, we have to learn to set realistic goals and create clear strategies that get us there. It's true what they say: when we fail to plan, we plan to fail.

We've already figured out effortless strategies to empty your barrel, and now it's about putting them into realistic timeframes and creating strategies to make them achievable.

So you can ask yourself: How many action steps are realistic for me to implement within what timeframe? How exactly do I plan to implement them? What do I need for the implementation?

Then think of each area you picked and ask yourself specific questions regarding the action steps, for example:

- How long do I want to follow the exercise plan?
- How often do I want to do my favorite activity?
- How much time will I need to work on changing my perception towards the stress factor?

4.2 INCREASING YOUR CHANCES TO PERSEVERE

After having set your goals and basic implementation strategy, use these three tips so that you can increase the chances of sticking with your back-health plan.

1. The first and most important thing is to increase your inner motivation because it's mainly your motivation that will determine whether or not you achieve a goal.

Basically, there are many ways to motivate yourself that work well, but some will work only for a short time, whereas others work longer. Generally speaking, our long-term chances of success are at their highest if we either love doing the activity so much that we can't wait to do it (we're usually in a "flow state" whenever we do it), or if it's something that's really important to us (so that it activates the Prefrontal Cortex which quiets down immediate desires in favor of a long-term goal). If we go after those intrinsically motivated goals, we also benefit from not being at the mercy of the psychological phenomena of the "licensing effect" which explains that people often want to treat themselves when they did something that's perceived as "good, "such as having that piece of cake after a hard workout.

If we feel compelled to do something, act out of a bad conscience, or need outer incentives to get motivated, we tend to "license" ourselves to compensate for our achievements. While we might empty the barrel with one behavior, we fill it up with the compensating behavior again. To get out of this circle and achieve long-lasting behavioral changes, we need to find what sparks our inner motivation.

While in the last chapter we already picked out the action steps that most inspire you and that you most love doing, adding meaning to them by looking for reasons why they're important to you will further increase the chances of your long-term success.

So, if we see enough benefits from doing the back-health plan, we'll increase our inner motivation, enabling us to put aside all doubts and excuses while getting us out of your comfort zones whenever needed. At this point, we won't have to be reminded or push ourselves to pursue those activities.

Whatever action steps you've chosen, try to connect them to everything that's important in your life! Ask yourself: How is doing these things helping me live to my highest potential? Just like in the Reason Determination section, think of every area of your life and connect it to what's most important to you in these seven areas:

1. professional
2. financial
3. family
4. physical
5. social
6. mental
7. spiritual

So for example, if your business is most important to you, ask yourself: How will taking care of my back health, my ergonomics, or my diet help me to get my business flourishing?

2. The second way to increase your chances to persevere is by committing to the challenge. For this there are three levels of commitment which have varying degrees of power. The first level is you. Since we only have to justify ourselves to ourselves, there's a great temptation to break that commitment. Nevertheless, it's the most important one because you will only successfully complete the challenge if you are convinced of it yourself. You can write your commitment to pursue the back-health plan for a certain amount of time on a piece of paper and hang it up in your bedroom to remind you of your commitment every day.

The second level is social obligation. Tell your friends, family, or followers on social media that you are participating in a new plan for your back health. This brings a lot of motivation because we don't want to have to disappoint our family and friends.

The third level is financial. The loss of money usually has a stronger effect than the gain. So here you could put money aside, which you donate or otherwise give away in case you don't keep up with your plan. The best motivational effect is when you combine several levels. For example, if you commit to your spouse to buy him or her a new TV if you don't meet your goals, you link the social to the financial level.

3. Lastly, thinking of what obstacles could come your way and how you could overcome them offers a great chance to implement the action steps with more certainty and self-efficacy. In the building industry, for example, people plan out a big building project by thinking about everything that could go wrong and putting contingency plans in place for each case. Why don't you do the same with your project for getting a sustainably healthy back and create your own project contingency plan? It will solidify your plans and definitely increase your convictions the plan is right for you.

To create your own contingency plans, think about each action step and what it takes to implement it. What obstacle could you face on the way to bring more ergonomics into your workplace, to do your favorite activity again, or to optimize your environment at home?

Now think of what you could do to overcome those obstacles. Could you get creative and build your own ergonomic workplace if you don't get the adjustable desk from your boss? Go sign up for a membership at the gym close by so you can jog on the treadmill whenever the weather is bad? Or buy a sleeping mask if your spouse doesn't like sleeping in complete darkness?

Thinking about those contingency plans will help you not fall back into the victim role whenever things aren't working out the way you expected.

4.3 TWEAKING THE PLAN IF YOU HAVE SETBACKS

Even if you planned it all out, increased your inner motivation, and thought of contingency plans, sometimes there can still be setbacks. You might feel more pain after the first time you did your favorite activity; maybe you didn't pursue your health plan even though you've been highly motivated; or maybe your friends didn't come to the dinner party you hosted. Those aren't necessarily bad things which prove that it all doesn't work, but rather they're just feedback that the path you've chosen wasn't 100% aligned with what's really most important to you, with your body's current capability to bear load, or with your friends' plans and priorities.

If you've had a setback, and the pain increases again, remember that slight irritations of the structures are normal after long inactivity and pain doesn't necessarily mean that something has to be "broken" again. Your nervous system may just be trying to protect you by descending amplification. However, since the nervous system sometimes just overreacts and our mind does the same by having catastrophic thoughts again, we can try to overwrite this pattern. Otherwise those thoughts can quickly lead us to give up, return to the victim's role, and try radical, short-term pain treatments that ultimately take us a step away from sustained back health.

But we don't want to downplay the pain either as it is real, but if we try to perceive it in a more neutral way, we can simply make changes to our approaches so that the warning system doesn't fire so quickly again. You now have enough ideas in several areas with which you can tweak your back-health plan. Above all, it might be necessary to consider the load management tips again.

4.4 PRACTICING GRATITUDE

Creating a gratitude list can increase your health and reduce your stress levels. When we're grateful for something, a beautiful feeling arises in us and our heart opens.

If we consciously try to give more attention to the things that work as we planned, we can increase our gratitude. If, for example, we focus on the fact that we're blessed to have a well-paid job after all, or that we are still able to go jogging despite all our joint degenerations, we can significantly increase our level of gratitude.

If we can also see how things that are supposedly not going so well also bring advantages and opportunities with them, we can be grateful for those. Even though this can be much harder because it requires deeper thinking, the gratitude we develop for our challenges can turn distress into eustress and empty our barrel significantly. I've learned to be grateful for my knee and back problems because I've become aware of all the advantages and possibilities they brought with them. This made it easier for me to find meaning in my challenges and to give up my role as a victim.

I encourage you to write a gratitude list because it will also help ward against the increased occurrence of distress and depressive moods. So list all things for which you're grateful in your life, and then every evening you add at least three new things you were grateful for that day.

4.5 GOING AFTER WHAT INSPIRES YOU MOST

You now have an idea of what an EFFORTLESS approach is. In the end, it's all about doing things that you can do effortlessly, that, when you stick with them, will create momentum. Those things can either be small and easily changed without much work involved, or something that includes more work but because it inspires you, doesn't feel like work. Even though the former approach can make a big difference for your pain immediately, the latter approach might empty your barrel even more because it increases your self-efficacy, joy of life, and self-worth.

If you make those small changes that make a difference in your pain, don't just sit back and think that was all that was needed, but go after the inspirational things as well. There might've been areas in which the action steps actually inspired you but you didn't see how you could implement them in your everyday life or you weren't really convinced that they would help you. But if the inspiration is strong enough, we're usually able to overcome those doubts and realize that following what truly inspires us, is actually more effortless than we thought. So, give yourself permission to also believe in your ability to go after those most inspiring things because that will help you empty your barrel long term. Going after things that truly inspire you will break you out of the victim role and push you out of your comfort zone.

So, go through all of the different areas again and look at which action steps you assigned the greatest value to with regard to the inspiration question and try to double check the doubts you had surrounding those action steps.

While in this book this concept relates to your back health, if you really understand it, you might also be able to apply it to other areas of your life. In the search for your ideal career path, for example, sorting out options by asking yourself the three questions of the EFFORTLESS method can help to pick the most effortless and inspiring option. Going after that option then helps keep the barrel empty as it will create eustress rather than distress.

4.6 MAKING IT AN EFFORTLESS HABIT

After picking your most effortless and inspiring things, finally think about which of those you could implement into your life as a habit or daily routine. In order to acquire a habit, we usually need anywhere between 21 to 66 days, provided we perform the activity daily. Since the back-health plan activities were effortless, you may be able to make them become habitual more easily and quickly, but only if you do so purposefully. A habit means that we do something without having to think about it and without major difficulties—that is, it's effortless.

Look at all the action steps in your back-health plan and pick the one action step that you want to make into an effortless habit. Of course, it should be an activity that's actually possible to do regularly. Is it your individual exercise plan, a stress management method that you plan to work with every day, or your favorite activity that you plan to do regularly from now on? But remember, always consider what's realistic for you and don't set your expectations too high right away.

4.7 YOUR BARREL, YOUR QUALITY OF LIFE

In this book, you've read that back pain is more complex than you likely previously thought. This can be overwhelming or confusing. In the end, dealing with the pain is quite simple. Keeping the barrel as empty as possible means your back health improves accordingly. And there's no right or wrong. You decide for yourself what empties your barrel best.

Perhaps it's the activities in the 10 EFFORTLESS categories, or perhaps something completely different that you just came up while reading this book. The most important thing is that you become attuned to your own body and decide for yourself what will help to empty your barrel in the long run.

Even though there might be approaches that have stood the test of time, ultimately the "right" sitting posture as well as the "right" sport or the "right" exercise doesn't exist for everyone. Every person and every back is individual.

I hope this book has given you the ability to make the "right" decisions for emptying your personal barrel. If you take responsibility for yourself and focus on mastering your back health in the long run, you will also empower other areas of your life.

Instead of going after immediate pain relief at all costs, try to focus on your quality of life that will increase the more you've emptied your barrel, even if the pain in your back doesn't completely disappear right away. And even if the pain comes back at some point, you now have enough strategies at hand for improving the condition of your back through some effortless action steps.

After my own herniated discs about 10 years ago, I couldn't find any effective strategies against the discomfort, so helping others to be free from back pain is a mission of mine. If only one thought, one tip, or one action step made a difference for you and your back pain, it would fulfill me and therefore empty my barrel as well.

So thank you for reading my book, and I wish you a life full of back health, vitality, and fulfillment.

BIBLIOGRAPHY

- Butler, S. (2013). *Explain Pain (2nd edition)*. Adelaide, Australia: Noigroup
- Cook, G. (2011). *Movement. Functional movement systems: Screening, assessment, corrective strategies*. Aptos, USA: On Target Publications.
- Demartini, J. (2013). *The values factor. The secret to creating an inspired and fulfilling life*. New York, USA: The Berkley Publishing Group.
- Gokhale, E. (2013). *No more back pain. Permanent improvement in 8 steps*. Munich: Riva.
- Goodman, E. (2016). *True to form: How to use foundation training for sustained pain relief and every day*. New York, USA: Harper Wave.
- Hitzmann, S. (2013). *The MELT method. A breakthrough self-treatment system to eliminate chronic pain, erase the signs of aging, and feel fantastic in just 10 minutes a day!* New York, USA: HarperOne.
- Cave, K. (2016). *Uexküll Psychosomatic Medicine. Theoretical models and clinical practice*. Munich: Elsevier.
- Fritzsche, K. (2020). P*sychosomatic Medicine. An International Guide for the Primary Care Setting*. Berlin, Germany: Springer
- McGill, S. (2015). *Low back disorders. Evidence-based prevention and rehabilitation (Third Edition)*. Champaign, USA: Human Kinetics.
- McGill, S. (2015). *Back mechanic. The secrets to a healthy spine your doctor isn´t telling you*. Ontario, Kanada: Backfitpro Inc.
- Osar, E. (2017). *The psoas solution. The practitioner's guide to rehabilitation, corrective exercise, and training for improved function*. Berkeley, USA: North Atlantic Books.
- Schleip, R. (2017). Fascia fitness. How to be Vital, Elastic and Dynamic in Everyday Life and Sport. Chichester, UK: Lotus Publishing.
- Sahrmann, S. (2001). *Diagnosis and treatment of movement impairment Syndromes*.
- Oxford, England: Elsevier.

ADDITIONAL RESOURCES

- www.drdemartini.com
- www.health.harvard.edu/plate/healthy-eating-plate
- www.pain-ed.com
- www.precision-nutrition.de
- www.retrainpain.org

CREDITS

Cover design: Annika Naas

Interior design: Anja Elsen

Typesetting: Guido Maetzing, www.mmedia-agentur.de

Cover photos: © AdobeStock

Interior photos: © AdobeStock, pp. 33, 36, 43, 67, 69, 72;
all other photos © Ramin Waraghai

Interior illustrations: © AdobeStock, pp. 18, 42, 65, 117, 145-148;
all other illustrations © Ramin Waraghai

Photographer: Juliane Mann

Managing editor: Elizabeth Evans